COMING
OF AGE ON
ZOLOFT

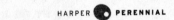

HARPER PERENNIAL

NEW YORK • LONDON • TORONTO • SYDNEY • NEW DELHI • AUCKLAND

COMING OF AGE ON ZOLOFT

HOW ANTIDEPRESSANTS CHEERED US UP,
LET US DOWN, AND CHANGED WHO WE ARE

KATHERINE SHARPE

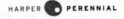

COMING OF AGE ON ZOLOFT. Copyright © 2012 by Katherine Sharpe. All rights reserved. Printed in the United States of America. No part of this book may be used or reproduced in any manner whatsoever without written permission except in the case of brief quotations embodied in critical articles and reviews. For information address HarperCollins Publishers, 10 East 53rd Street, New York, NY 10022.

HarperCollins books may be purchased for educational, business, or sales promotional use. For information please write: Special Markets Department, HarperCollins Publishers, 10 East 53rd Street, New York, NY 10022.

FIRST EDITION

Designed by Fritz Metsch

Library of Congress Cataloging-in-Publication Data is available upon request.

ISBN 978-0-06-205973-4

12 13 14 15 16 ov/rrd 10 9 8 7 6 5 4 3 2 1

For my parents

Everybody's youth is a dream, a form of chemi

—F. SCOTT FITZGERALD

CONTENTS

Introduction   xi

1. The Diagnosis   1
2. A Short History of Medication   25
3. Starting Out   53
4. Decade of the Brain   85
5. I've Never Been to Me   109
6. Two Red Chairs   135
7. Flight of the Dodo Bird: Evaluating Therapy   165
8. Quitting   193
9. Converts   225
10. The Next Generation   251
11. Coming of Age   279

Acknowledgments   299
Notes   301
Bibliography   307

INTRODUCTION

One afternoon late in the summer of 1998, I found myself sitting on the long front porch of a weathered student house in Portland, Oregon. I was nineteen years old and had just returned to town to start my second year of college. The porch I was sitting on belonged to the house that would be home that year to my good friend Kate. I had spent the day helping her move in, relaying loads of clothing, books, and LPs from her car, across the yard, up a staircase scuffed by decades of similar use, and into her new room. At 5:00 P.M., exhausted, we flopped onto the row of mismatched seating that looked out over the cracked, gray street.

Moving off campus was a sophomore rite of passage at our school, and I considered Kate's snagging a room in this particular house to be a promising social development. Her new housemates included some of the students on campus I'd looked up to most the year before—smart, fashionable, confident women who seemed as advanced and distant to me then as I remembered high school seniors seeming when I was in eighth grade. As they filtered in and slowly took their own seats around us, I stretched in my thrift-store lounger and smiled. Simply sharing their porch with them felt glamorous, like a good omen for the year to come.

Late-afternoon sun gilded the floorboards, as our conversation meandered through the familiar topics of professors, classes, boys, and books. Kate headed inside to organize her room, and Lauren mixed a pitcher of Amaretto sours for those who were left. And then the thing happened that has fixed this afternoon in my mind for more than a decade. Casually, and in the abstract, someone mentioned antidepressants.

The comment sent a ripple through me. I had been taking an antidepressant since the year before, when a series of anxiety attacks had led me to the student health center, where I'd quickly been diagnosed as depressed and given a prescription for Zoloft. Medication seemed to have helped; the billowing dread that had come upon me during my freshman fall had dissipated, and I'd finished out the year with good grades, friends, a boyfriend, new interests. Still, I felt uneasy about my chemically assisted recovery. There was something creepy about taking a mind-altering drug each day, and thinking of myself as a person with a mental disorder was dispiriting in its own right. Aside from a few close friends, I hadn't told anybody I took them; I figured other people would find the fact as off-putting as I did myself.

I still don't know what it was that made me open my mouth that day. Maybe I was lulled by the sunshine, the strange drink, or the urge, in such exalted company, to say something that would call attention to myself.

"I take those," I blurted and instantly looked down at my hands, wondering whether I'd just effected my own social excommunication. When I managed to raise my eyes again, though, I saw that heads up and down the row were nodding slowly.

"I do too," said Helen.

"They put me on Prozac last year," Lauren added. And on we went. There were seven girls on that porch. Every single one of us, it turned out, was or had been on antidepressants.

In the moments afterward, we looked out toward the street, where a patch of weeds cast a long shadow across the pavement. "This is really weird," somebody said, and the rest of us mumbled assent.

AS I COLLECTED myself in the silence, I felt two things at the same time. The first was a wave of relief so large and pure it almost knocked me over. All year, taking medication had made me feel uneasy. The pills imparted strength and calm, but they also raised tough questions—*Am I crazy? Will I need these forever? Am I really myself when I take them?*—that I could neither answer to my satisfaction nor successfully push from my mind. Learning that I wasn't alone in using medication soothed the sense of alienation that had been the pills' most notable side effect. If people as poised and admirable as Kate's housemates could also take antidepressants, maybe there was still hope for me.

But if learning that I had so much company on the antidepressant bandwagon was comforting in one way, it was disorienting in another. I had been taught to think of antidepressants as a treatment for depression, which I understood as a real illness, something rare and serious. The fact that all seven of us could be taking medication strained the limits of my sense of probability. Were we all, in some meaningful way, mentally ill? Or were antidepressants being given out not for true depression but precisely for the ordinary angst that I'd been told was so different from it? If we all had this experience in common, why had we not found out about it until now? I felt a little dizzy, and newly suspicious. What exactly was *happening* here?

Before that moment, taking antidepressants had felt like the most intimate and personal thing in the world to me. It was still personal, of course, but I began to see then that it was also more than that. Medication was individual, but also social; it was part of our stories, but equally part of the story of a time and place. In a way that I didn't yet fully understand, our lives had intersected with something larger than themselves.

It is strange, as a young person, to realize that you have lived through something that can be considered a real historical change, but that's exactly what we had done. When I was a child, in the early 1980s, taking psychiatric medication was decidedly a fringe phenomenon. Prozac came onto the market in 1987, the year I was eight. The first member of a family of drugs called SSRIs (for "selective serotonin reuptake inhibitors"), it quickly became the leading edge of a psychopharmaceutical revolution. Throughout the 1990s and 2000s, Americans grew ever more likely to reach for a pill to address a wide variety of mental and emotional problems. We also became more likely to think of those problems as a kind of disease, manifestations of an innate biochemical imbalance. Depression, social anxiety, obsessive-compulsive disorder, and the like went from being strange clinical terms or scrupulously hidden secrets to constituting acceptable topics of cocktail party conversation—talk that was often followed up by chatter about the new miracle drugs for despair.

Statistics bear out the sense of changing habits. Antidepressants began to climb steadily in popularity after Prozac's introduction, eventually becoming a truly mass phenomenon. By 2005, SSRIs had surpassed blood pressure medications to become the most-used class of drugs in America,[1] with 10 percent of adults taking them in any given month.[2] By 2008, that figure had bumped up to 11 percent.[3] While they were becoming part of the fabric of American life, psychopharmaceuticals also became, with much greater frequency, a part of American youth: in 2008, 5 percent of adolescents aged twelve to nineteen took an antidepressant.[4] The same year, another 6 percent of twelve-to-nineteen-year-olds used psychostimulant medication for ADHD.[5]

Nothing has changed since that moment on the porch, I sometimes think, except that I'm not surprised anymore. Antidepressants are part of the story of my generation, an invisible but very real strand woven through our collective experience. Psychiatric medication saturated the country during our childhood and adolescence, and for many of us, the involvement became personal. In our twenties and thirties now, with birthdays that fall from the mid-1970s to the start of the 1990s, we are members of the first generation to have literally grown up on psychiatric medications in significant numbers.

And sometimes those numbers still overwhelm me. Antidepressant use saturates certain populations more than others, which may help explain why antidepressants have often struck me as being even more ubiquitous among my peers than the above figures suggest. Women take them at higher rates than men, a difference that emerges in early adolescence; a recent survey found that 16 percent of women use antidepressants, compared to 6 percent of men.[6] White adolescents are more than five times as likely to use an antidepressant than black adolescents, and more than twice as likely as Latino adolescents,[7] racial disparities that also hold true for adults.[8] Personally, I can't remember the last time I shared the topic of this book with a group of more than three twenty- or thirtysomethings without eliciting someone's own medication story, often from the person I least expected. Not long ago, I was talking to a male friend, age thirty-five, who exclaimed, only half in jest, "I've never *known* a girl who wasn't on antidepressants!" I must have come a long way from Portland, because I knew exactly what he meant.

THIS IS A book about what it's like to grow up on antidepressants. It attempts a faithful description of an activity that has become remarkably common—using antidepressants as a teenager or young adult—but still engenders intense, complicated, and often conflicted feelings, both in the young people who do it and the adults who are involved in their care. Advertisements and reductive media stories often portray antidepressant use as simple. Depression is a disease "like diabetes," the story goes, and the appropriate treatment is equally straightforward: find a doctor, locate a pill, take it, and be well. Further soul-searching about it isn't just unnecessary, it's likely to be counterproductive. But the truth is that even when the medications work just as they are supposed to, taking antidepressants is an experience that can feel profound. Rightly or wrongly, antidepressants command powerful emotions; they can lead people to examine their deepest assumptions about themselves and the world.

It is also an experience that can be substantially different for a young person than it is for an adult. Ever since the early 1990s, much of our cultural conversation about antidepressants has revolved around questions of selfhood. Adults who take antidepressants have been known to worry whether the medication is altering their habits, their proclivities, or their outlook on life—whether it is in some way changing the very people they are inside. Conversely, adults who are happy with their treatment often speak of antidepressants as facilitating a return to authenticity; they say that medication "turned me back into my old self again." Indeed, the notion that depression distorts the true self and that antidepressants merely restore what was there all along has often been invoked against the fear that by taking antidepressants, we might somehow be betraying our true natures.

But that belief in particular is one that people who start medication young cannot fall back on. Worries about how antidepressants might affect the self are greatly magnified for people who begin using them in adolescence, before they've developed a stable, adult sense of self. Lacking a reliable conception of what it is to feel "like themselves," young people have no way to gauge the effects of the drugs on their developing personalities. Searching for identity—asking "Who am I?" and combing the inner and outer worlds for an answer that seems to fit—is the main developmental task of the teenage years. And for some young adults, the idea of taking a medication that could frustrate that search can become a discouraging, painful preoccupation.

When I first began to use Zoloft, my inability to pick apart my "real" thoughts and emotions from those imparted by the drug made me feel bereft. The trouble seemed to have everything to do with being young. I was conscious of needing to figure out my own interests and point myself in a direction in the world, and the fact of being on medication seemed frighteningly to compound the possibilities for error. How could I ever find my way in life if I didn't even know which feelings were mine?

For me, as for many members of my generation, the process of growing up became linked to the practice of taking medication and thinking about mental disorder. In aggregate, my antidepressant story is not dramatic. By the standards of the sensational medication memoirs that I began to track down and devour in college, in an attempt to better understand what I was going through, it is positively vanilla. After the moment on Kate's porch, though, I began for the first time to think that my story might have an interest and a relevance of its own—not because it was so very unique, but precisely because it wasn't. Before that day, I'd been interested in tracking my experience on medication for personal reasons, but afterward I redoubled my efforts; I literally started to take better notes. I ended up using antidepressants for most of ten years, and the story of that unfolding relationship—during which my perspective on myself, on medication, and on the nature of health all changed significantly—is part of what structures this book.

Realizing that other people my age used antidepressants too whetted my appetite to hear their own stories. I wanted to know whether others felt as ambivalent about antidepressants and about the diagnoses that came with them as I did, whether medication had raised the same difficult questions for them as it had for me. The handful of casual conversations that I had about these topics over the years always fascinated me. In order to write this book, I interviewed forty people, ranging in age from eighteen to forty, about their own experiences growing up on antidepressants, and I corresponded by e-mail with about a dozen more. Talking to them revealed common themes in the experience of using psychiatric medication as a young person and turned up many points of contact as well as divergence from my own story. Their words and points of view are incorporated throughout the book.

Part of the reason why the moment on the porch stayed with

me for so long was the sheer force of the relief it brought me to connect, in person, with other people whose experiences mirrored my own. Though times have changed and it's hard to imagine, today, any young person believing that they're alone in taking a psychotropic medication, my research confirmed that medication use is still not something that people talk about with each other in-depth or regularly. But there is understanding to be gained in such conversations; partaking in stories of one another is one of the purest and most elemental forms of comfort available to us in our sped-up, surface-happy world. When I conducted the interviews for this book, a number of the people I talked to thanked me. They told me that they didn't speak about these topics very often, and that they were excited to hear what others had to say. One of my highest hopes for this book is that it will in some small way replicate the effects of that moment on the porch in Portland. I hope that people who take or have taken antidepressants will find these stories recognizable, thought provoking, and ultimately affirming, and that friends and family will feel helped to a greater understanding of an experience that can be hard to put into words.

I also hope that this book will contribute something to a debate that has unfolded over the course of the psychopharmaceutical revolution. There is no question that the last twenty-five years have seen a great change in terms of how we conceive of emotional and behavioral problems, which we've moved decisively towards classifying as biochemical disorders. There is a lively cultural argument going on now about whether that's been good or bad. Critics of the shift contend that the "medicalization" of what were once regarded as negative feelings or nuisance parts of life has harmed us, that mental disorder is now overdiagnosed and psychiatric medications are overprescribed. They argue that we've moved beyond fighting legitimate psychiatric illness and have begun to wage pharmaceutical warfare on ordinary sadness—a war that has given undue power to "experts," lined the pockets of pharmaceutical companies, and left the rest of us feeling enfeebled, more ill than we truly are. Proponents argue that the revolution hasn't yet gone far enough. They claim we've made headway in reducing the stigma surrounding mental disorder but that there's work yet to be done, and contend that emotional problems are still, on balance, undertreated. This grand debate about the value of our turn to medication marches forward though a series of more practical ones. Prominent figures argue about whether antidepressants are "truly" effective, or merely fancy placebos, and the question about a possible link between antidepressants and suicidal behavior in children and adolescents is still open.

This book won't settle those debates, but it does speak to them. Twenty-five years after the introduction of Prozac, we are still collectively attempting to figure out what an appropriate use of medication would look like, in our culture and in our individual lives. We are trying to figure out what our sadness and pain mean—if they mean anything at all—and when they attain the status of illness. We're trying to figure out when to turn to pills, when to go another route, and how we might be able to tell. This book isn't a polemic or a self-help title. It can't tell you whether you need help or what kind to get. But it does believe that good answers to the big questions about medication are likely to proceed from careful attention to the actual experiences of the people who have faced them. Stories like the ones collected here may help us to a more realistic assessment of what antidepressants can and can't do, when they are a good idea, and when the detriments might outweigh the benefits. And it is in that spirit that I offer the story of my own decade of antidepressant use and how it intersected with my path to adulthood, and the stories of many of the forty-plus people who spoke to me about the same thing.

1 | THE DIAGNOSIS

To describe how I got started on antidepressants, I could reach way back. I could tell you about my earliest memories, or give background on my parents or even my grandparents. But the best place to start is the summer of 1997 in Arlington, Virginia, a hot one even by the standards of the Washington, D.C., area. In the suburbs, the air itself often seemed to sag around street level, holding the smells of grass clippings, car exhaust, and barbecue in its thick embrace. People moved slowly, and once in a while someone made the old crack questioning the wisdom of our founding fathers' decision to build their capital city on a malarial swamp.

That summer I was seventeen and, like other seventeen-year-olds I knew, I used my car to get places. I had access to an ancient, bright orange Volvo sedan that had belonged to my grandfather, which I loved almost as fiercely as the act of driving itself. Most days, I drove to the coffee shop where my best friend, Sarah, and I both worked. Early-morning drives to the shop were the best, before 6:00 A.M., the streets empty, the sun already blazing up like a pink rubber ball over the rolling hills of Arlington. After work I drove to Sarah's house, took myself on shopping errands at strip malls lined with big-box stores, or went to the parklike cemetery to read or write. Sometimes at night we would drive just for the sake of driving. We'd aim Sarah's Cutlass Ciera down the George Washington Parkway, which runs alongside the Potomac River. I liked the way the lights of the city's bridges seemed to float like jewels in the water, the humid night air pouring in the windows, the feeling of the road ahead all clear.

SCHOOL HAD ENDED in the middle of June, an occasion marked by a graduation ceremony complete with tears, hugs, yearbooks to sign, and a pool party afterward. My parents surprised me by giving me a camera as a graduation present, and in the weeks that followed I used it to take pictures of every familiar thing: my mom's tuna fish salad, glistening with red onion; my father standing in the kitchen, drinking coffee; my younger sister at the diner, saying something funny, mouth open, a cigarette in her hand, her blue eyes big and bright. I added older pictures I'd taken of friends—Huey, Josh, Ellie, and Anne, even a couple of my ex-boyfriend, Scott—and pressed them all between the pages of a small photo album to take away to college at the summer's end.

It was hard to imagine a world past school and Arlington. Some people hate high school, but I hadn't. The small, public magnet school I'd attended since sixth grade had suited me well; at best, it had felt like a real community, and I'd been that rare kid who is happier and more social as a teenager than as a child. I had even picked my future college, a small liberal arts school in Oregon, because its culture reminded me of my old school in many ways. Still, the idea of really leaving H-B Woodlawn and the life I'd known behind made me feel sad. Sad, and though I tried to block it out with excitement, more than a little scared.

At first, fear and anxiety came in the guise of nostalgia. I decided to spend the summer commemorating everything I'd loved about the past six or seven years. I would revisit every place I'd ever been to, go to every restaurant or park or coffee shop I'd ever liked, one last time, return to the scene of every milestone or event or fight that had seemed important. I would soak it all in thoroughly, fix it in my mind forever, revel in the bittersweet intensity of a phase of life nearing its end. And somehow, I imagined, that would make me ready to face what was next.

Scott had broken up with me the week after graduation. He walked from his house down the block over to mine, and we sat on my parents' gray couch and talked about how it wasn't working out. In one sense, the breakup was no big deal. We had barely even seen each other all spring. When I was honest with myself, it was easy to see that it was right for it to end. We had drifted together during early senior year when we were both working on a school play. But we had always been an odd couple. Scott was straight edge, I wasn't; he did wholesome things like improv theater and Model United Nations, while I read Beat poetry and sneaked cigarettes in the parking lot behind the school. Beyond a shared sense of mild outsider status, we had never understood each other well. By dumping me he was only giving voice to what was already obviously true.

Still, the breakup created a space that seemed to attract all kinds of negativity into itself. My mind began to curdle, and my nostalgic agenda for the summer started to take on a nihilistic edge. I didn't want to do anything new or meet anyone I didn't know already. *What's the point?* my mind would ask. *We're all just leaving anyway*. Abstractly, I knew that leaving home for college meant a fresh start, a rebirth. But most of the time I couldn't see past the part that felt like dying, everything I'd known collapsing in on itself like an exploded star.

On the night of my eighteenth birthday, I walked into the darkened playing field behind my high school, a few blocks from my house. The air was warm and sultry, shorts and T-shirt weather even well after dark. Grass and clover tugged at my ankles. I sat on the split-rail fence, held my face in my hands, and cried. Whatever life was, I wasn't sure I was up to it. Normal things had begun to feel unbearably poignant: the last time I hauled a heavy garbage bag of coffee grounds out to the Dumpster in the sweltering parking lot behind work, the familiar action, never to be repeated, almost reduced me to tears. The future seemed unimaginable; I felt like I was about to be pushed into the Coliseum with a bunch of wild animals. Was I ready? Could I possibly be ready? Would I ever do the things I wanted to do, would I ever be normal? Would anyone ever love me? Dear god, would I ever get laid? It all seemed terribly impossible to visualize.

When I look back from today on my mood that summer, it's not hard to see reasons why I felt unsettled. I think that I was suffering from lack of daily structure, and a straightforward fear of leaving home, probably compounded by a lack of self-confidence. But from the inside, it didn't seem clear or understandable at all. I didn't feel afraid of school, exactly; I felt flawed—in some way so strange, complete, and unique that I couldn't even fathom it, let alone do anything on my own behalf. I exaggerated in my mind how wonderful high school had been. The truth was that after all those years I was sick of it. I needed new challenges and new people. But most of the time I had no access to those yearnings. All I felt was a penetrating fear of loneliness, and deep grief for all that I would leave behind.

In the evenings I consigned my fears to the pages of my journal. In purple pen, I wrote: *I'm scared shitless of going to college, but this is such a big subject it's hard to get started. I go crazy. But how to be specific? Wild moods. Frantic, or complete apathy.* And a few days later: *It's when I think about all the things left to do in life—big and small things equally—that I think I can't go on. Everything makes me want to throw up today.*

SARAH DIDN'T UNDERSTAND my frame of mind. She seemed to be flourishing: working at the coffee shop, getting to know all the patrons, dating one of them, and then another. She couldn't be happier to finally be free of high school. With her long brown hair and her nose ring and her newfound aura of indomitability, she looked beautiful.

"You need to relax," she said to me one afternoon. We were sitting in her bedroom, me on the bed, Sarah in a desk chair beneath her enormous Pink Floyd poster. "This is a summer for having fun," she continued. "We did it. We're on top of the heap. We're going to college. This summer is our *reward*."

"I know," I said. "I know! I shouldn't be taking things so seriously." Sarah's point of view sounded reasonable and wise; I just couldn't make it stick in my own case.

"We need to get you some fun," she said. "You should have a summer fling."

"What's the point of a summer fling? We're all just leaving."

"That's *exactly* the point," she said, taking a sock-ball from the dresser and throwing it at me. "You're hopeless!"

"I'm not hopeless!"

"Yes you are," she said, rolling forward in her desk chair, then hauling her body upright. "Come on. Let's go get some home fries."

YET FEELING BAD wasn't the whole story of that time. Looking back, it almost seems as if there were two summers, simultaneous and nonintersecting. There was the summer I felt bad in, and there was the beautiful, intense summer. The summer in which Sarah and I rocketed down the George Washington Parkway in her car after midnight, blasting the Smashing Pumpkins, deep in the crazy love that only high school best friends can have for each other. The summer in which I devoted my afternoons to writing a novella that was meant to weave my observations about the people and places I'd known in high school into a kaleidoscopic whole. There are bubbly, excitable entries in my journals that parallel the angry, mournful ones. In August, I went to see Scott in a production of *A Midsummer Night's Dream*, and we talked afterward and it felt good, like closure. It *was* excellent to be through with high school. At certain moments, that feeling that Sarah talked about would settle, drift down on us like valedictory snow. We'd made it. Hail to us.

Was I depressed? It seems strange to say, but that is not a question I asked myself then. If I had graduated high school in 2007 instead of 1997, it seems inevitable that I would have asked myself the question, or that someone else would have asked it for me. How would I answer? No—I wasn't depressed, exactly, because depression is supposed to go on for weeks, unbroken, and no feeling I had that summer lasted for any length of time. Were my moods abnormal? It's hard to say. I did seem to be taking the transition harder than my friends were. But then, I'd always been serious, romantic, tightly wound. Maybe I was just living these things in my own way.

Anyway, in the end, what can you do? The summer got late, and then later. One day while I was stopped at an intersection in my mom's car a song came on the radio, with a gravelly voiced man singing about how *"I hope I was everything I was supposed to be."* As the light turned green, a guy in the oncoming lane leaned his head out of his window and shouted, "Don't cry!" But it didn't matter. Days passed, I finished up at work, Sarah went off to college in Iowa, and a few days later my time came too.

REED COLLEGE SITS in a neighborhood of one- and two-story houses in the southeast quadrant of Portland, Oregon. Architecturally, the campus presents a jumbled mix of stately collegiate Gothic buildings and angular 1970s affordabilia. At the top of a hill rising East there's a Safeway and a discount store, a bar and a restaurant, a post office and a Plaid Pantry. There is nothing distinguished about the area, but I loved Portland from the moment I set eyes on it. Douglas firs rose from the hilltops, giving the whole city the look of an Alpine theme park, and the air felt fresh and energized, scrubbed clean by its trip across the Pacific. On a clear day I could catch sight of the distant, snowy mass of Mount Hood, poking from the horizon like a giant's chipped tooth.

At the beginning of freshman orientation week, my father helped me move into my new room. He made a few runs to the store with me for things like coat hangers and laundry detergent, gave me a big hug, and then he was gone.

What was it I had been so afraid would happen? After a few

nights, I could hardly remember. From the moment I set foot in Portland, my mood had turned around with a speed and decisiveness that shocked me. The transformation was so swift that it was almost embarrassing, the edifice of gloom I'd built with such painstaking care all summer tumbling down flimsily under the first volley of new people and new things.

For the first week at school I ricocheted around the campus like an atomic particle: meeting, bonding, splitting, repeating, releasing energy in all directions. I found a girl to go thrift-shopping with on Eighty-Second Avenue. I met Darlene and Rob, who had been friends together in high school in Arizona. A boy from a nearby hall got a crush on me, but I wasn't interested. I got a crush on a senior who played the cello, but it didn't last. Some people from my dorm and I went to a party up the street, at a punk house with a keg in the backyard and a kitchen decorated with six-foot-tall signs salvaged or stolen from the meat department of a supermarket. A reddish stop-motion filmstrip of a seed sprouting into a plant projected in a loop on the bathroom wall while a four-piece rock band played loud in the living room.

On the third day, I was fiddling with the combination dial on my student mailbox when I bumped elbows with a girl who was doing the same thing. She smiled and shook her head. "How do you work these damn things?" she asked. I said I didn't know either. "I'm Kate," said the girl, stretching out her hand. "I guess your box is right above mine." Kate had long, deep red hair, straight bangs, and a trace of Texas in her voice. The moment I looked into her kind hazel eyes, I felt sure that of all the people I'd talked to, this one was going to be a friend.

"I'm Katherine," I said. "Hey—do you want to go to the Paradox and get some coffee?"

"Okay." It was that easy. How could I have fretted so much about ever finding human connection? One could no more avoid it than step in between raindrops.

THROUGH KATE, I met everyone else who mattered. She lived in the oldest building on campus, a beautiful Gothic dorm shot through by a crazy system of hallways that reminded me of the tunnels in an ant farm. I began to spend most of my free time there, with Kate, her hall mates, or the boys who lived in a triple nearby. Classes started, and freshmen began to troop together in large packs to weekday-morning lectures. We talked about them afterwards, and about our professors, picking apart their foibles the way people pick apart celebrities. The shared excitement felt good. I had never been in a place where knowing things wasn't at least potentially a liability. In high school there had been little pockets where being engaged in what you were studying was an asset, something that could bring you closer to other people rather than marking you off as strange. But this was a whole new league of play, and I began to want nothing more than to rise and distinguish myself in it. I felt so relieved to realize that I hadn't been wrong about Reed. I liked it as much now that I was there as I had thought I would on college night in the high school gymnasium the year before.

A couple of weeks in, I made friends with one of the boys from the triple. Brendan had curly brown hair that grazed his shoulders, and he wore perfectly rumpled white button-down shirts. He had gone to boarding school, which meant that he'd skipped right over the homesickness part of college and already had considerable experience having fun in an institutional setting. Most evenings he held court in Kate's social room, talking and spinning stories for anyone who passed by, his loud, bleating laugh bouncing off the walls and reverberating in the next hall over. He dressed up like F. Scott Fitzgerald for Halloween, claimed to know what brand of cigarettes Kurt Vonnegut smoked, and promptly worked out five ways to get onto the roof of the building. He thought I was funny, and I found him completely enthralling.

Brendan quickly became the person on campus I most hoped to run into, the one for whom my eyes scanned the quad and the student union with the greatest diligence. He had a college radio show on Saturday mornings, and I used to get up early and sit with him while he was on the air. The studio was just a room in the basement of one of the dorms, furnished with a couch whose arms had been rendered hard and shiny from years of rubbed-in food and hand oils. But when I sank into its cushions and listened to Brendan play the oddities he'd harvested from the station's groaning shelves of records, I couldn't imagine a place in the world I'd rather be.

The fonder I grew of Brendan, the more I realized that not all of my friends saw him the same way. Ted said that Brendan had teased him ruthlessly while he, Ted, was high and Brendan wasn't. Jessica said that Brendan seemed smarmy, but I couldn't understand what she was talking about. Brendan was amazing. Being around him felt amazing. I wanted to be with him all the time. I had a desperate crush on him, of course, but there was more to it than that. I wanted to be *like* him. The things about myself that I wasn't so sure about—the seriousness, the deliberation, the tendency to worry—were nowhere evident in him. Where some people saw arrogance, I saw a boy who was carefree, at home in the world and in his skin in a way that I would have given almost anything to be.

Midterms came, a week of intensely concentrated stress but also a bleary-eyed camaraderie that affected the whole campus and made the time pleasant in its own delirious way. I'd stay in the computer labs until two or three in the morning, with Kate or whomever, working on papers under fluorescent light until our minds went swimming in the undersea murals of seaweed and turtles and fish to which some campus wag had added stumpy cigarettes and thick-rimmed glasses in precise black Sharpie marker. On one of the nights of the reading period, I took a study break with Brendan. We walked to the far end of campus and sat on a log in the undergrowth behind the theater building. We were on the log, and then we were off it, rolling around in the ivy, kissing frantically. I took my glasses off and, after a few minutes, realized that I couldn't find them. I began patting down the brush all around us, casually at first, then wildly. Brendan sat on his heels and watched impassively until I pulled them out of the vines—a rudeness that registered, but not as decisively as I wish it had.

On the hall where Brendan lived there was a room so tiny that the residence life office didn't even assign it to anybody. At one point, Brendan's hall mates had picked the lock. They decorated the space with a bong, some pornographic playing cards, and a few condoms, and dubbed it "the sex room." A couple of nights after the log incident, I don't remember quite how, Brendan and I ended up in the sex room. We definitely didn't have sex there, not even close. We fooled around for a while and then fell asleep with our clothes on. By the time I woke up, just after dawn, I was shivering with cold. Brendan was nowhere to be found, and something felt obscurely but undeniably wrong.

When I try to remember the next few days, I get an image of breaking glass: they have that quality of crash and splintering. I finished work, turned in papers, and slept fitfully. I looked for Brendan everywhere, but when I finally did manage to track him down, he acted as if a stranger had invaded his body. He spoke in monosyllables, as though I were someone he didn't know, or particularly care to start knowing; he directed his words in the general direction of my face while managing to avoid my eyes completely. He didn't break up with me or talk about what had happened (what *had* happened? I felt unsure of anything anymore), but it seemed clear that from his point of view, our friendship, and its whiff of romance too, was decisively and unceremoniously over. I walked away, feeling light-headed. Later someone told me they'd seen him hanging around campus with another girl, whom I knew just vaguely, and who was beautiful. My friends told me I was better off without him, that there were dozens of worthier guys all around us, but I couldn't hear them; I felt as if I'd been cut open, my organs removed, and my body filled with something as hard and heavy as gravel.

My last conversation with Brendan happened a day or two before I was supposed to fly home for fall break. I got up early on that Saturday morning and followed the instructions I'd written myself about how to take the bus to the light rail to the airport. I felt tired, hungover, and strangely deflated. The past nine weeks had been hectic, I thought, and maybe it was a good idea to take a few days in Arlington to slow down.

———

DESCRIBING WHAT COMES next feels unsatisfying any way I try it: I can't make the facts seem to match up with my reaction, and so it seems that I must be exaggerating or leaving something out. But it happened just like this.

My flight home had a layover in Saint Louis. On the carpet near my gate, I sat in a pool of light that streamed in through big plate-glass windows, and scribbled in my journal. My face was puffy from crying so much. A different girl would have been furious with Brendan, but I didn't feel anger, just the sting of rejection, the creeping, hemmed-in sensation of shame.

"It looks like you're writing a 'Dear John' letter," said a voice. I looked up. It was a TWA staff member in a blue polyester uniform. She sounded hearty and amused.

"A what?"

"You know: 'Dear John, by the time you read this, I'll be gone . . .'"

"Oh yeah. Well, I guess I am, kind of."

I tried to enjoy being at home. Fall was usually my favorite season in Virginia. But my mind couldn't seem to find a comfortable position. I felt sad and agitated at the same time. The happy letters home, dated just weeks earlier, that my parents had taped to the refrigerator door seemed to have been written by someone else—a silly, naive person I didn't know.

One morning, maybe my second at home, I decided to take my mother's bicycle out for a ride. I wasn't a frequent rider, but going for a spin seemed like something to do that would get me out of the house, a way to discharge the strange, irritable energy I'd noticed in myself. Soon I was following "BIKE ROUTE" signs down sleepy streets that led toward a paved trail. A few brown oak leaves waved, like hands in gloves, high up in a sky of perfect

East Coast blue. I could see that the day was beautiful, but I was still waiting for it to produce in me the happiness that I expected from crystalline October days in Virginia. What I felt instead was that biking seemed harder than I remembered. I could feel my breath ripping unevenly in and out of my chest. I tried to shift down, but the gears seemed to behave exactly the opposite of the way I expected them to, and it got even more difficult to pedal. I was on familiar streets in a familiar neighborhood less than two miles from my home, but for some reason I began to panic. Or worse than panic: I felt a wave of despair rise, ripple through my body, and escape as heat from the top of my head. My stomach turned over. I didn't want to be there, and a moment later I knew that I didn't want to be anywhere. Merely living suddenly just seemed too hard, too undignified. The burn in my thighs, instead of meaning healthy exercise, felt like an emblem for the pain of life in general, a sickly reminder of every struggle to come. I mounted a small hill, and the gears crunched; the chain went slow and then slower until all my effort to push it forward came to nothing. The wheels ground to a stop and I thought, *I can't do this! I'm so pathetic. I don't know why I'm even trying.*

The bike fell to one side and I got off. Underneath the blue sky, I was dwarfed by oak trees and surrounded by orderly cottages on a nice suburban cul-de-sac. In the calm of the middle of a weekday, the surroundings seemed almost creepily indifferent, like the set of a horror movie. Not far off, the highway rushed softly. I felt a sensation of life speeding away from me on all sides. The world seemed so distant, so impossible to understand. I saw a pile of mulch, a scrum of bamboo, and clapboard siding. I knew the surroundings were friendly, but felt as out of place as something that had crash-landed on a strange planet. I held the unwieldy bulk of the bike in one hand, and wiped with the other at the tears that were sliding down my face. I tried to calm my breathing and, dizzy with shame, hobbled the bike away from the scene as gingerly as if I had fallen and skinned my knee.

FORTY-FIVE MINUTES AFTER I'd left, I quietly returned home. My mother was standing in the kitchen with her back to me, washing a sink full of dishes. "Oh!" she said cheerfully, turning around. "You're back soon!"

Though there are few legitimate uses for this English word, I think it would be accurate to say that I wailed as I fell into her soapy arms. "What's the matter?" she asked, fear spiking her voice up a few notes. She held me back at arm's length, scanning my body for a visible wound.

"I'm sorry," I said, sniffling and shaking, teary and confused. She looked me in the eye, and I flinched, as though her face were a flashlight exposing every hidden imperfection in me. I opened my mouth and blurted out the first thing that seemed true. "I just. Really. Don't like myself right now."

My mother waltz-marched me backward to the gray sectional sofa in the family room. As I remember, I spent most of the rest of the week on that sofa. The violently bad feelings subsided, leaving a residue of dullness and fear. I felt all right when I stayed in my nest, wrapped in afghans and watching TV, but I was terrified of what would happen to me when I had to return. It seemed as if all the strength and enthusiasm of the past nine weeks were gone, and I was right back to the worst of where I'd been over the summer, feeling unfit for the world and not up to the everyday tasks other people take in stride. These feelings seemed connected to Brendan, at one end, but they quickly spun off into something bigger, a dread without boundaries. I wondered what was happening to me. Was this the same malaise from the summer; had it been lurking for me all this time? Had my nine weeks of happiness at school been real, or were they the deviation, and this awful state my true baseline all along?

I wasn't writing in my journal at the time, so I can't consult it. Years later, though, I asked my parents what they remembered from my days on the gray sofa, and what they'd made of what was happening then.

My mother told me that she'd thought I was heartbroken. She said she knew how badly I had wanted to fall in love, that she'd watched me try and fail back in high school to reap what every song and movie and book for teenagers holds out as the pinnacle of a young life. She had been there when I was in tenth grade and a group of boys that I and another girl were close to had turned away as sharply and bafflingly as a school of fish, cutting us off completely. Maybe she even perceived that there might be, in this recent rejection, an echo of that one, which made it doubly painful. From what little I had told her about Brendan, it was easy for her to imagine that I had been disappointed and was taking it hard. And if there was something irrational and over-the-top about my mood that week—well, both she and many of her friends, she said, had breakdowns of one kind or another during college, and went on to lead normal lives. She hated to see me unhappy, but she thought I'd persevere. Sooner or later something good would happen, and it would bring me up with it.

My father took a different view, one that was rooted in his own experience. For most of my life, even before I was sure what the words meant, I had known that my father thought of himself as depressed, or depressive. The year I was eleven or twelve, he started taking an antidepressant, and I still remember the positive difference it made in him, and in the emotional climate of our whole household by extension. Long before the idea gained popular currency, my dad believed that he suffered from a genetically determined tendency to biochemical depression, and the fact that medication worked for him solidified his view that that was the case. And so, where my mother saw a case of teenage Sturm und Drang, my father saw biology asserting itself. He had worried a lot over the years about the possibility that he'd passed the depressive parts of his genetic code on to his daughters, and what was happening to me that year seemed to confirm his worst fears. When I asked him about it, he remembered that when he'd dropped me off at campus in August, I looked pale and wobbly. Nine weeks later, he'd seen me walk off an airplane with tears on my face. What was he supposed to think? These two visions made a deeper impression than the perky letters sent in between. He thought I probably needed medicine.

And what did I think? I felt close to my dad, but I'd never seriously considered the possibility that I might be depressed in the same way that he was. In high school I'd understood myself to experience mood swings—which went up as well as down, thank you very much—but that seemed like my sovereign teenage right. I didn't know anyone my age who used antidepressants; medication seemed to belong to a world of grown-up feelings and choices that had nothing to do with me. And maybe that's the way I wanted it. At some point in high school I had started to think of myself as a writer, an identity that meant to me then, among other things, that feelings were important. Emotion was the raw material from which everything else was going to proceed, I believed, and anything that might blunt or change mine would have seemed inimical to my vague but dearly-held ambitions. On the other hand, this new state I was in scared me deeply. College felt like a fast-moving river. There was no safe time-out place to crawl into, nothing comparable to the gray sofa at home. I felt like I had to be poised and under control at all times, and I was ready to consider just about any solution that presented itself.

Toward the end of the week, my parents and I sat in conference on the deep cushions of the sofa. I remember my mother telling me, half-jokingly, that I didn't have to go back to college if I didn't want to. If it was a gambit, it worked: even in my state, I could tell that nothing good would come of brooding on my parents' couch forever. Instead, the two of them asked me to promise that when I returned, I would immediately make an appointment for myself at the school's Health and Counseling Center. We agreed they'd get me the help I needed, whatever that turned out to be.

THE PLANE LANDED. I caught a bus back to campus and flipped on the lights of my dorm room. The Pacific Northwest drizzle had begun; it would continue seemingly without end until May. My room didn't look so homey or exciting anymore, but I was grateful to be able to hang out in Kate's. Decorated with beeswax church candles and big pieces of fabric, and suffused with Kate's comfortable and comforting presence, it was the closest thing on campus to an oasis.

During those first days back, I felt torn between wanting to maintain my dignity and a wish to tell someone what I'd been going through, to try to ask for a little extra patience or care. One night shortly after classes had begun, Kate and I walked across the soccer field at the back of the campus, on our way to the Plaid Pantry for study food: Cup O' Noodles, Slim Jims, or a pint of Häagen-Dazs. Kate asked me how I was, and I chose that dark, soft moment to begin crying again. "Not that good," I whispered. Saying the words made me feel destabilized. It was like dipping a hand beneath the surface of the fear that seemed to always be there, since just before the start of fall break, like an icy ocean that any casual stimulus—a song, a kind word, a harsh word, it hardly mattered—would plunge me down into, until I lost my breath among the floes.

"Oh darlin'," said Kate, her Texas drawl the spirit of unfussy compassion. She put her arms around me. I can still see her small hands with their chipped cherry red nail polish. I swabbed at my eyes with the back of my sleeve, feeling silly but relieved—ashamed to be demanding this extra attention but wordlessly grateful for a loving friend.

THE HEALTH CENTER at Reed College is a mossy cottage in an out-of-the-way spot near the center of campus. From the outside, it looks like a building where the heroine in a Brontë novel would live; it has that kind of weedy, wild charm. I had been inside once or twice already to stock up on the free generic medicines they gave out in single-dose paper packets: ibuprofen, aspirin, acet-aminophen, cough drops, and the red nasal-decongestant pills that people took to stay awake while writing papers in these, the years before Adderall. I'd seen the free condoms and lube that rested in bins decorated cheerily with construction paper and yarn, as though enough kindly wishes on the part of the Health Center staff could make sex not just physically but emotionally safer too, and the weathered copies of *Prevention* and the Reed alumni magazine that sagged comfortably, like banana peels, on its waiting room tables.

I signed my name and student number into a ledger, and a nurse at the intake window asked me what I was here for. I crowded up, trying to create a seal between myself and the student in line behind me. "Counseling," I whispered, as softly as I could, then took a seat and waited for what was next.

"Katherine?" The woman calling my name had dark hair and a serious face. She introduced herself as Sam and led me upstairs to a consultation room with a sloping ceiling that reminded me of my childhood bedroom. Sam closed behind us two doors hung in a single frame ("The rooms are soundproofed for privacy," she explained) and gestured for me to take a seat in one of two over-stuffed armchairs. She sat down in the other one, crossed her legs, balanced a pad of paper on her top thigh, and looked at me. I dug my fingertips into the plushy arms of the chair and looked right back at her.

"So," Sam said. "What brings you here?"

I took a deep breath and let it out again. "Where should I start?"

"Start wherever feels natural," she said.

"Okay." My lip trembled, and then I began, floodgate-style. I told her about the summer, about worrying all the time, about coming to school and feeling better. I told her about the boy and the crush and the bike ride and falling apart and spending a week in a ball on the couch. I told her how a similar thing had happened when I was fourteen and tried to baby-sit for the first time, how I'd managed it then by not babysitting anymore, but it didn't seem so easy just to avoid love and college, did it?!

I helped myself to one of Sam's tissues while she wrote notes down on her little pad. As I watched her hand move across the paper I felt an odd mix of relief and humiliation.

Sam guided our conversation to more straightforward things. She asked if I'd been sleeping (yes, to excess); whether I'd been eating (to tell the truth, I didn't have much of an appetite); whether I was getting my classwork done (sure, classwork was about the only thing I was getting done).

She asked me some questions that, even in my state, I could tell were meant to separate the truly crazy people from the merely, well, whatever I was. "Have you ever thought about harming yourself or others?" *No.* "Do you ever hear things that other people don't hear?" *No!* "Do you ever feel like . . ." She paused, just for a beat, as though even she were slightly embarrassed by the question to come. "Do you ever feel like maybe just not wanting to live anymore?"

Oh boy. "Well," I said carefully. I tried to explain it to her. It wasn't like I was some kind of suicidal *maniac.* But were there times lately, in the middle of long prickly afternoons, when it occurred to me what a relief it might be if there were a way to simply not, you know, exist? Yeah, there were times like that.

"In psychiatric circles," said Sam, "that's what we call passive thoughts of death."

She asked me about my family, and I told her about how my father was still taking his antidepressant faithfully. I told her about my sister, still in high school, and her new group of troubled-seeming friends. I told her about my mom's propensity to worry, and the stories I'd heard about the time when my grandmother took to her bed for a week, issuing instructions to her children about how to make their own breakfasts.

Sam nodded, smoothed a piece of dark brown hair behind her ear, and looked at me again. Then she reached for another, smaller pad from the desk behind her.

"I think you have depression," she said carefully. "I'm going to write you a prescription for Zoloft. I'm also going to go downstairs and find some samples so you can get started right now."

She left the room. I looked at the clock; we'd been talking for about twenty minutes. I felt like an eggshell, a brittle teacup. I felt like she'd told me to sit still and wait because it was her professional opinion that if I made a move in any direction I might break into a million pieces. *Right now!" That's how bad she thought it was*, I told myself.

Zoloft.

Oh, god.

I imagined a heavenly tattoo needle coming down from space to etch the scarlet letter D right into my skin.

SAM RETURNED TO the room with five or six small cardboard boxes printed in blue, green, and white: free samples of Zoloft. She thrust them into my hands, and I put them in my messenger bag, where for the rest of the day, the tiny pills rattled around in their bottles like dried beans.

That evening I locked the door of my side of the dorm room, took out the boxes, and opened one. Out slid a plastic vial and a tissue-thin sheet of patient information, folded in a tight crimp. It had a diagram of the Zoloft molecule and a section on "pharmacokinetics." The pills themselves were sky blue, capsule shaped, lovely. I knocked one into the palm of my hand, tilted my head back, swallowed, and waited.

2 | A SHORT HISTORY OF MEDICATION

For a week or more I didn't notice anything different, just the mood I'd returned to school in, wrapped around me like a heavy blanket. Back on campus I settled into a quiet version of my old routines, but I often felt exhausted, as if once-simple tasks required an effort that was almost impossible to muster. I craved the company of other people, in a diffuse way, but I felt unprepared for the rigors of conversation: my responses to things had to be dredged up from a great depth, it seemed, and inevitably arrived a couple of beats too late. Hiding out in Kate's room presented a solution. In the afternoons, we sprawled out on her floor with our translations of Plato and Lucretius; around 5:00 P.M., we'd carry back something greasy from the dining hall, to eat in the safety of the dark patch of linoleum between Kate's and her roommate's beds.

But if I was dull and flattened in one way, I also felt revoltingly attuned in another. Out in the world beyond my few safe places, everything seemed like too much. I felt as if my skin had been removed, leaving me transparent and totally unprotected from the minor radiation of everyday life; every word or glance or impression ripped right through me. If you have ever cried at a movie or a wedding, you know what it's like to be grasped by a sense of life so big and mysterious that you can't contain it; it overwhelms you in an instant, and the excess feeling, all that can't be comprehended, leaks out in tears because it has nowhere else to go. When I was depressed I felt that way about everything, except instead of love and beauty, the excess was sadness, futility, and pain. It was wedding-tears precisely inverted: the presentiment of loss and impermanence that gives happy moments their luminous quality was the central fact, and the presumptive existence of happiness and goodness elsewhere, far away, was what made life seem so unbearably sad.

And so I did cry, at everything. It was as if some emotional pitch detector inside me had broken. Everything meant something, but the meaning was always the same. Even inanimate objects, animals, and trees talked to me about suffering. Sitting by the plate-glass windows in the dining hall, watching a squirrel pick its way across a telephone wire, and wobble, and recover: this was the stuff of high tragedy. In reality, this period couldn't have lasted for more than a couple of weeks, but in my memory it seems to stretch on forever—a strange little eternity in which shedding tears became a basic bodily function to be fulfilled regularly and by rote, a little pick-me-up squeezed into my hourly, between-class visits to the end-of-row stall in the ladies' room on the first floor of Vollum Hall.

And then one day, the Zoloft started to work. At first all I felt were some of the side effects I'd been warned about: headache, dry mouth, a new and different kind of sleepiness. A day or two later I stopped crying, just like that. The tragedy I'd been watching came to an unexpected end, and I collected my coat and walked out into the street, surprised to find myself thinking about something other than life, death, the infinite. Not only was I free not to think about them, but for the first time in weeks they didn't seem any more interesting than anything else: plans for the weekend, say, or conjugating Latin verbs. In the mornings, my stomach rumbled for breakfast.

At first, I studied the medicine's effects on me with interest. In one sense, they were hard to define. I wasn't sure how much to credit my improvement to the passage of time, or to being back at school—which, with its many pulls on my time and attention, was an environment much less conducive to brooding than home was. But even allowing for some of that, I feel confident that the Zoloft helped. The change was just too swift and decisive to be completely explainable in any other way.

After a few more weeks I decided that Zoloft was having at least one strange effect. I began to feel less anxious—about everything: not just free of my recent panic, but calmer in every single realm of my life. It was as if some persistent, low-grade undertone of alarm, something so constant that it had never fully registered before, had fallen silent, announcing itself by its absence for the first time. I noticed it most in relation to work; on Zoloft, it became easier than ever before to close the books, say "Good enough," and declare myself done for the night. But I also felt looser at parties, less self-conscious in the moments before class. I enjoyed the new way of being, but it was peculiar too, and even distressing in its own way. I never thought that I had loved that old anxiety, but it had felt like me. What would I be if not driven? More weeks passed and gave the lie to my immediate fear—that I wouldn't work as hard, and my grades would suffer—but even afterwards, I held onto the worry that some deep and necessary inner balance might have been shifted, and that the consequences, not that I would ever fully know them, would be bad.

AS I SETTLED more firmly into feeling better that fall, I began to get curious about my new diagnosis and new treatment. I had an informal sense of what depression was, of course, but I realized, as I thumbed through what I knew, that my understanding was far from complete. I wanted to know what I had, where my medicine had come from, and how exactly it was fixing whatever had gone wrong inside my brain.

I attacked these questions in a way that is typical for me: I started to read. The "Prozac"-titled memoirs just beginning to appear on the front tables at Borders were good for a first course, and by spring semester I was deep into dense university-press tomes with names like *Neuronal Man* and *A Primer of Drug Action*. I found this private research soothing. The idea of having depression made my life feel out of my hands in a way it never had before, and trying to master the topic seemed to go partway towards restoring the missing sense of control.

Sam had upped me to a stronger dose by then, the pills not blue but a pale, pleasant yellow, a color that would have looked right on the walls of a guest bedroom in the country. Some nights I held the capsule in my hand for an extra moment and wondered to myself, *What is this thing? What in the hell am I doing?*

If you start to read up on depression, one of the first things you'll learn is that the history of your condition is sprawlingly complex. Part of the reason, it seems, is semantic—depression, or states that we might recognize as such, has been described by doctors and philosophers and ordinary people alike over thousands of years, in terms that sound similar but also subtly different. In the second century B.C., the Greek physician Hippocrates described patients suffering from an illness he called "melancholia"; they exhibited despondency, loss of appetite, excessive fear, and difficulty falling asleep. Spiritual writers in England during the Middle Ages spoke of a state known as "acedia" or "wanhope," which was a disease in one sense, and a sin in another. As the Parson in Chaucer's *Canterbury Tales* lectures his fellow travelers, the evils of wanhope include "outrageous sorrow," a crushing sense of guilt and self-loathing, and a dull heaviness "in body and soul," which if left unchecked can lead to despair of salvation and eventually suicide. Centuries later, the Romantic poets described melancholy as a frame of mind, a mood state that could be exquisitely painful but also beautiful in its own way, a badge of refinement and a source of insight. Freud, like the Greeks, used the term "melancholia"; he meant it to describe a psychological illness that felt like grief, which a person could succumb to after losing an important relationship or possession, or suffering the violation of a cherished value. If melancholia seemed often to descend out of nowhere, he argued, that was because the losses involved were generally subconscious.

Depression, in other words, was like an octopus, sliding through history—recognizable but slippery, undulating and changing shape, its many tentacles in many different pies. It had been described as a physical ailment, a spiritual condition, a temperament, and a reaction to loss. It had been portrayed as normal—something we all go through, to varying degrees—and as profoundly strange, a form of madness. If it was, in some sense, the same thing in all these permutations, you would also have to concede that it was a rangy, diverse, unwieldy thing indeed.

All right, I thought as I read. This is all very interesting. But surely we've come up with something more satisfyingly specific in our day. Surely we have settled by now, against these quaint theories, the question of what depression *really* is?

We certainly had a definition that sounded crisp and definite. In making her diagnosis, I learned, Sam would have relied on a book called the DSM-IV, for *Diagnostic and Statistical Manual of Mental Disorders, Fourth Edition*. The volume, published in Washington by the American Psychiatric Association, compiled information on all known mental disorders and their symptoms; newspaper articles often referred to it as the "Bible" of psychiatry. The DSM defined depression as the presence "most of the day, nearly every day," for two weeks or more, of at least five from a list of nine symptoms that included "depressed mood," "loss of interest or pleasure," unintentional weight loss, sleep disturbances, psychomotor agitation or retardation, fatigue, feelings of worthlessness, diminished concentration, and thoughts of death or plans for suicide.

That sounded straightforward enough. And according to the DSM criteria, I *had* been depressed, or would have been if my symptoms had rolled on unchecked for a few more days. But where had the DSM definition come from? My attempt to figure that out set me on a path of reading and research that eventually led all the way back to the 1950s. Following it gave me a sense of both how new and unprecedented our current understanding of depression was, and how closely and recursively its rise had been tied to the development of modern pharmacology itself. I learned that though our contemporary definition of depression was specific, it wasn't, in all its particulars, necessarily any more empirical than Hippocrates's working definition of melancholia (or, for that matter, any more verifiable than a medieval cleric's views on wanhope). In short, the story of the Prozac revolution wasn't a tale of crisp scientific breakthrough. Instead it was a case of science and culture pulling each other along together, our concept of a complicated illness shifting to correspond to our most promising means of treating it. The story of the invention of modern antidepressants and the story of the invention of depression as we know it go hand in hand.

PROZAC WAS BROUGHT to market in the 1980s, but if it had a family tree, the year "1952" might be carved in near the base of the trunk. On July 5 of that year, a front-page article in the *New York Times* called attention to a medical mystery unfolding on the tuberculosis wards of two New York–area hospitals. Doctors conducting a clinical trial of an experimental T.B. drug called Marsilid had reported that while the new medication didn't appear to help the patients' wounds heal, it did seem to have caused a remarkable transformation in their spirits. The doctor in charge told the *Times* that Marsilid induced "a state of euphoria," which mellowed over a few weeks to "a normally optimistic instead of a depressed attitude."[1] Though Marsilid seemed to make people healthier, no one could figure out exactly why; tests showed that the patients' infected tissues were just as clogged with tuberculosis germs after treatment with the drug as they had been before it.

I don't think I'll be giving away too much if I tell you that Marsilid turned out to be an antidepressant. But you might think it strange that the doctor didn't make that leap, even though he used the word *depressed* while gushing to the *Times* reporter. In fact, nobody speculated that Marsilid might be used as a drug for a mental disorder. The *Times* article closed with a lukewarm observation that since the early effects of Marsilid sometimes resembled a "mild narcotism," the medication might eventually find a niche as a treatment for drug addicts trying to kick the habit.[2]

To us today, it seems self-evident that antidepressants would be successful drugs, and valuable ones. After all, depression is everywhere. The World Health Organization identifies depression as the leading cause of disability worldwide.[3] Researchers estimate that depression costs tens of billions annually in lost productivity.[4] The way that Marsilid was received in its day reveals how much our beliefs about depression have changed over the decades. It didn't immediately occur to the researchers that they had discovered an antidepressant, largely because, sixty years ago, people thought of depression very differently from the way we do now.

It's not that they didn't recognize it. In fact, psychiatrists of the time were familiar with two different kinds of depression. One they called "endogenous depression" or "vital depression," which referred to a profoundly depressed state that was thought to be due to biological causes.[5] Endogenous depression was characterized by insomnia, loss of appetite, psychomotor retardation, and sustained feelings of intense despair: people who had it weren't just sad, they were afflicted in a patently physical way.[6] But endogenous depression was thought to be extremely rare. Psychiatrists also recognized a more common and often (though not always) less severe type of depression, which they called "depressive neurosis." Depressive neuroses were not thought to be biological or biochemical in nature, but rather the result of normal psychological processes, like conflict and loss.[7] This everyday depression was spoken about casually, as a diffuse mood state that could arise for any number of reasons, but not as a specific, well-defined ailment of its own. Back then, most depression was more adjective than noun: it was a way you felt, not something you "had" or "were."

Endogenous depression was believed to be so rare that pharmaceutical companies didn't even think there would be enough of a market to support a drug for it.[8] (Depressive neuroses, while very common, weren't considered an appropriate target for drug development; since they were thought to be a product of normal psychological functioning, coming up with a drug to treat their causes would have been an idea that just didn't compute.[9]) But in the period of intensive pharmaceutical research and development that followed the end of World War II, interest in drugs for mental illness had begun to stir. Thorazine, the first commercially successful psychopharmaceutical, was discovered in 1950 in France; it was an "antipsychotic" drug used to treat schizophrenia.[10] At the time, most people in the industry assumed that the next profitable psychiatric medication would be yet another antipsychotic.[11] And that's just what scientists at the Geigy corporation in Switzerland were looking for when, almost at the same time as T.B. patients in New York were cheering up under the influence of Marsilid, they invented an experimental compound called imipramine. Imipramine proved hopeless as an antipsychotic. In clinical trials, it made schizophrenic patients boisterous and hard to control. But it certainly seemed to have some effect on mood. If the drug could tip schizophrenic patients into mania, some of the researchers reasoned, maybe it could help bring endogenously depressed patients the energy they needed to get well.

The exact origin of the decision to test imipramine on a tiny group of people with endogenous depression is hazy. But the trial, carried out in 1955 at a small country hospital in Switzerland, produced astonishing results. The very first patient recovered from her delusional depression within six days, and the next two also showed vivid improvement.[12] Before the trial period was over, the head researcher wrote to imipramine's manufacturer to state his opinion that the company had discovered a true drug for depression.

This time the psychiatric community took notice. In 1958 imipramine, which had been given the brand name Tofranil, went on the market in Europe as an antidepressant.[13] By this point, some psychiatrists in America had become interested in Marsilid's antidepressant properties (an early champion, Dr. Nathan Kline, called Marsilid a "psychic energizer"), and it had also gone on sale as a treatment for depression. But neither drug exactly flew off the shelves, largely due to the belief among psychiatrists that endogenous depression was extremely rare. (To give you an idea of the tone of the discourse, an April 1957 article in the *Times* hailed the antidepressant Marsilid as a breakthrough treatment for the "unreachable, severely depressed mental patient."[14]) A few years later, Marsilid was pulled off the market when it was found to cause jaundice in a small number of cases.[15] Imipramine, which was the first of what are known as "tricyclic antidepressants," for their three-ring molecular structure, is actually still on the market in the U.S. and Europe; numerous studies have shown it to be equally or more effective than Prozac.[16] Antidepressants had arrived, but the antidepressant revolution was still a few decades off. Before it could hit with full force, our ideas about what depression was would have to undergo their own transformation.

———

IF YOU CLOSE your eyes and try to imagine scientists inventing a cure for an illness, you probably assume that they have at least a pretty good idea of how the disease works, and that they use that understanding to take aim at specific targets in the body. That's more or less how I assumed the story of the development of antidepressants would go. But in the case of depression, my presumption ran precisely backward. Antidepressants were invented by accident—twice—and scientists drew conclusions about the nature of the illness by investigating the action of the drugs.

Neuroscience is still a young discipline, and it was even younger in the early 1950s. During that decade, researchers in search of a challenge applied themselves to the problem of untangling how the two new classes of antidepressants worked. The first mystery was that while drugs in Marsilid's family and drugs in imipramine's family were both effective treatments for endogenous depression, they appeared at first to perform very different actions inside the brain.

Through a series of ingenious experiments, researchers discovered that while the two types of drugs do work in different ways, they lead to virtually the same end result. Each drug causes higher concentrations of the neurotransmitter norepinephrine to be present in the synapses—the tiny spaces in between the nerve cells that make up the brain, across which brain cells communicate with each other by chemical signals.[17, 18] Drugs in imipramine's family, the tricyclics, do this by blocking the re-absorption, or reuptake, of norepinephrine from the synapse back into the nerve cells around it. Drugs in Marsilid's family, which came to be known as "MAO inhibitors," or MAOIs, do it by dampening the action of an enzyme that breaks down certain neurotransmitters, norepinephrine included. MAO inhibitors also boost brain levels of another neurotransmitter, serotonin.[19] Later research confirmed that tricyclic antidepressants do so too.[20]

Once scientists knew how the antidepressants worked, it was just about impossible to resist drawing up some new theories about what depression was. In 1965, a psychiatrist named Joseph Schildkraut pulled all that was known about antidepressant action into just such a theory. He used a process of simple reasoning backward: the known antidepressants, he observed, worked by raising the level of biogenic amines (a class of compounds that includes norepinephrine and serotonin) in the brain. Depression, he concluded, would therefore seem to be related to a deficiency of these same compounds—in other words, a chemical imbalance.[21] Schildkraut's ideas were known as the "amine hypotheses," and the *American Journal of Psychiatry* paper in which he introduced them went on to become one of the most cited in the history of the field.[22] "Thanks to Schildkraut," reads his 2006 obituary in the *Times* of London, "it was generally accepted that depression is a medical illness and that many mental disorders are related to imbalances in chemicals in the brain."[23]

In the 1960s, multiple types of each antidepressant went on the market. Nardil, Pamelor, and Elavil joined the other treatments in psychiatrists' arsenals. And psychiatrists did begin prescribing them to their most severely depressed patients. By 1987, about 1.8 percent of Americans purchased an antidepressant each year. That's not nothing, but it's hardly the explosive proliferation that would begin in the 1990s. Antidepressants might have remained a relatively specialized treatment, and the amine hypotheses just another piece of wonky scientific knowledge, lodged deep within its field. After all, endogenous depression was rare. Companies that made antidepressants didn't expect them to be big sellers, and they weren't. But changes were about to take place that would allow Schildkraut's amine hypotheses to take root and grow, subsuming the old distinction between endogenous and neurotic depression, and ultimately becoming one of those big ideas that seems to take society by storm.

WHEN SCHILDKRAUT WAS coming up with his amine hypotheses, the dominant framework in American psychiatry wasn't biochemical but psychoanalytic. During the 1940s, 1950s, and 1960s, most people who had nonpsychotic mental problems and could afford to pay a professional for help would have gone to a psychoanalyst with a more or less Freudian orientation, who would have understood their problems as some variety of psychological reaction and would have treated them with talk therapy.[24] Psychiatrists and the educated public alike assumed that most mental disturbances, even serious ones, were the result of intrapsychic processes involving inner conflicts and subconscious desires. Neurotic depressions and the like were understood as disorders of the emotions, but not diseases as such; in fact, Freud had used the term "neurosis" specifically to refer to a mental problem that was primarily psychological and not the result of any structural or functional problem in the brain.

It's hard to appreciate now how thoroughly ingrained psychoanalytic ideas had become. It was true to the extent that Nathan Kline, a famous American psychiatrist who tried to popularize antidepressants in the 1950s, first described those drugs' effects in *Freudian terms*: he hypothesized that MAOIs increased a person's vital energies by reining in the ego, which was responsible for keeping in check the primal, libidinous id. By freeing up a burst of raw power from the id, Kline said, the medication would whet a person's appetites for food, sex, and stimulation of all kinds, leading to a feeling of joyfulness and well-being.[25]

But by the 1960s, the psychoanalytic "establishment" was, as powerful incumbents will, attracting its share of criticism. Frustrated patients began to grouse that psychoanalysis was expensive and time-consuming. The technique didn't always seem to produce a marked improvement. And it was notably bad at helping the people who needed help most, people with schizophrenia or other psychotic illnesses. (Indeed, reading about psychiatrists' attempts to use the "talking cure" on its own to heal patients with severe mental illness is a poignant experience, and one that can put any critique of modern psychiatry into perspective.) Some people blasted analysts for being arrogant, always ready to blame a patient's failure to improve on that patient's subconscious "resistance," rather than on the shortcomings of their own method.[26]

Also, beginning in the 1950s, medications began to compete with talk therapy for the first time. These weren't antidepressants, which hadn't become popular enough to make waves, but prescription drugs meant to alleviate the symptoms of neurotic anxiety. Miltown, launched in 1955, was the first prescription antianxiety drug. In 1960 it was joined by Librium and Valium, members of a new drug family called the benzodiazapenes. Originally marketed to ease the strains of corporate life for hard-driving businessmen, "tranquilizers" turned into a phenomenon. Some estimates claim that by the mid-1970s, about 15 percent of the adult population of the United States was using them.[27] According to one apocryphal story, early demand for the pills was so great that ransacked drugstores were forced to hang out signs that read: NO MILTOWN TODAY.[28] Eventually the tranquilizers' popularity made them an object of mass cultural awareness, discussed and debated and joked-about in their era in much the same way that SSRIs have become in ours.

On the one hand, the tranquilizer explosion made psychiatry even more prominent and more influential. The availability of an easy fix for a common mental problem brought many new cases out of the woodwork, and demand for psychiatric services increased. On the other hand, tranquilizers could be read as a challenge to the psychoanalytic psychiatry of the day. They could be, and often were, prescribed by ordinary doctors rather than by expert psychiatrists.[29] And while no one presented tranquilizers as a true cure for anxiety or anything else—their effects lasted just a few pleasant hours, and then you had to take another dose—they did seem to make an end run around the psychoanalytic method. Why spend long years analyzing your problems when you can pop a pill and watch them melt away?

By the 1970s, the backlash against psychiatry had intensified. Psychiatrists became the butt of criticism from the countercultural movement, which saw them as rigid and authoritarian. In 1975 Miloš Forman released his film version of Ken Kesey's antipsychiatry novel *One Flew over the Cuckoo's Nest*, to critical acclaim. Two years earlier, a psychologist named David Rosenhan had humiliated the profession by performing an experiment in which perfectly healthy people presented themselves at mental hospitals, acting completely normal besides reporting that they had heard a voice saying the word "thud." The subjects were admitted, diagnosed as schizophrenic, and held, often for weeks and sometimes against their will; Rosenhan had his results published in the prestigious journal *Science*.[30] Many psychiatrists watched unhappily from the inside as their specialty threatened to descend into a national joke. Psychiatry, it seemed clear to many, needed to rehabilitate its image and bring itself in line with the times.

Some of them located the problem within psychiatry's comparatively unscientific nature. Psychiatry is a medical specialty, and all psychiatrists have MDs. But psychiatry had long been seen as something like the redheaded stepchild of medicine. Unlike other doctors, psychiatrists didn't perform surgeries or look at germs under microscopes; instead, they sat all day and *talked* to people. Plenty of analysts liked the subjective, interpersonal nature of their work just fine; for many, psychiatry's humanistic bent was what had drawn them to it in the first place. But an increasingly energetic group believed that for psychiatry to find its way again and regain the respect of the public, it needed to become more rigorous and empirical, more like other branches of medicine. They wanted their discipline to ease out of its tweed jacket and slip into a white lab coat.

A group of these reformers, mostly based at Washington University in Saint Louis, got control of the American Psychiatric Association committee that was charged with revising the *Diagnostic and Statistical Manual of Mental Disorders*. First published in 1952, the DSM was meant to classify all known mental disorders, in order to aid psychiatrists in their process of diagnosis.[31] To date, the book hadn't carried a lot of weight in the field. The second edition, from 1968, which was the one up for revision, is a pamphlet slim enough to be read from cover to cover in an afternoon. Its words illustrate the psychoanalytic leanings of American psychiatry at the time. For instance, here's how my condition in the fall of 1997 would have looked in DSM-II:

300.4 Depressive neurosis

This disorder is manifested by an excessive reaction of depression due to an internal conflict or to an identifiable event such as the loss of a love object or cherished possession. It is to be distinguished from *Involutional melancholia* (q.v.) and *Manic-depressive illness* (q.v.). *Reactive depressions* or *Depressive reactions* are to be classified here.[32]

The language about "reactions" comes from Adolf Meyer, a psychiatrist active in the 1920s and 1930s, who did much to package Freud's ideas for an American audience. Conditions that would now gain someone a prescription for Prozac were seen by Meyer as maladaptive responses to stressful circumstances, not as illnesses in a biological sense. (Ironically, it's Meyer who proposed using the word *depression* instead of Freud's term, *melancholia*; he thought that the latter word implied a level of scientific understanding that we simply didn't possess, while *depression*—which now sounds like the more scientific designation—was appropriately colloquial.)[33] Meyer's thinking fills DSM-II.

The group at Washington University overhauled DSM-II radically. DSM-III, which they unveiled in 1980, was 494 pages long to DSM-II's 119. (The trend has continued: DSM-IV, released in 1994, had ballooned to 886 pages, and DSM-5, due out in 2013, is expected to be even longer.) It contained more than two hundred categories of illness. Its tone was completely different too. The brief and impressionistic descriptions of mental disorders from DSM-II had been replaced by long checklists, meant to lead to better standardization of diagnosis. The authors of the new DSM were concerned with the fact, which had recently come to light, that different psychiatrists would often apply different diagnoses to the same individual. DSM-III endeavored to take the guesswork out. If a patient met a certain number of criteria from the list, he or she had the illness—end of story.

Most significantly, DSM-III stripped away all talk of "reactions" and "neuroses." Its introduction notes tartly that the new manual reflects "an increased commitment in our field to reliance on data as the basis for understanding mental disorders."[34] Since there were no data supporting the idea, for example, that depression was caused by an inner conflict or an excessive reaction to loss, that language was cut. The new manual didn't put any other causal theory in its place; in general, it remained much more concerned with the "what" of mental illness than the "why." But by clearing away Freud's legacy, DSM-III left the field wide open for a new theory to gain hold. And the scientific, medical tone established by DSM-III perfectly suited Schildkraut's very scientific-sounding amine theory of depression. In that hypothesis was a way of thinking that harmonized with psychiatry's ambition to shed its humanistic past and enter the fold of modern medicine.

MEANWHILE IN LABORATORIES in the United States and Europe, research and development work on antidepressants was continuing at its old sleepy pace. In 1972, an Eli Lilly scientist named David Wong and his group in Indianapolis synthesized a molecule that, they realized, inhibited the reuptake of serotonin from the synapses of the brain. But like the original discoverers of Marsilid, they didn't immediately realize that the new drug could be an antidepressant.[35] Though Schildkraut's amine theory mentioned both serotonin and norepinephrine, most of the neuroscience research on depression to date had focused on norepinephrine.

The Lilly company considered marketing its new compound as a blood-pressure medication (serotonin is present not just in the brain but also in the body, where it's involved in the expansion and contraction of blood vessels). But eventually clinical tests showed that the drug possesssed antidepressant properties, and it went on the market as Prozac in late 1987.

As best I can tell, no one expected Prozac to be a blockbuster drug. But it is clear that this new antidepressant emerged into a very different climate than the one that had greeted Marsilid and Tofranil thirty years before. The language of "neuroses" had been all but expunged from the new DSM, and the "scientific" and data-driven tone it had tried to establish was taking hold. The powerful figures in psychiatry were, increasingly, people who were in favor of seeing *all* mental problems as being ultimately biological in nature. The rise of the "biomedical model" of mental illness, which holds that mental disorders like depression are discrete physical diseases with biological causes, had begun— and Prozac would help it to prevail.

Another recent change made the time ripe for Prozac to succeed in a way that earlier antidepressants hadn't. Between the 1960s and the 1980s, the tranquilizers had gone out of favor. In 1971, the FDA censured tranquilizer manufacturers for marketing their drugs as treatments for the stresses and strains of everyday life, rather than as a remedy for any specific disease.[36] By the end of the decade, stories about tranquilizer addiction had begun to appear regularly in the press, and the public's love of tranquilizers started to turn into fear and ridicule. For the time being, Americans with minor mental problems were left without a go-to medication.

Prozac was soon followed by other drugs in its family. The

SmithKline Beecham company coined the term "selective serotonin reuptake inhibitor," or "SSRI," to describe Paxil when it came out in 1993.[37] Soon the term was applied to the whole class of drugs, which grew to include Celexa, Zoloft, Luvox, and Lexapro. "Selective" meant that unlike earlier antidepressants, the drug targeted only serotonin, not serotonin and norepinephrine both. The selectivity was supposed to be a selling point, the idea being that a more targeted drug would cause fewer side effects. Interest in norepinephrine's role in depression gradually faded away. (Only to return: like imipramine, the antidepressant Effexor, introduced in 1993, inhibits the reuptake of both norepinephrine and serotonin, leading some people to call it a serotonin-norepinephrine reuptake inhibitor, or SNRI. Other SNRIs include Cymbalta and Pristiq.)

The antidepressant explosion had begun. As usage of the new drugs stepped up, the biomedical model of mental illness gained currency, as the psychoanalytic model had done before it. Pharmaceutical companies spent millions of dollars on initiatives to educate people about depression; these invariably drove home the message that depression is a chemical imbalance best treated with a drug that acts on chemicals. (As I write this, language on the Zoloft website reads, with a weird mix of precision and vagueness: "Today, it's widely understood that depression is a serious medical condition. Scientists believe that it could be linked with an imbalance of a chemical in the brain called serotonin. If this imbalance happens, it can affect the way people feel."[38]) In college, I signed up for a psychopharmacology course offered by a new hire in the psychology department; in it we learned about reuptake, looking at diagrams of the lobe-like ends of neurons, with little particles of neurotransmitters bouncing in the clefts between them. Years later, Zoloft's manufacturer, Pfizer, would launch an advertising campaign that featured homey-looking drawings of the same thing. The first frame pictured two nerve cells, not treated with Zoloft: hardly any globs of neurotransmitter between them. It even *looked* sad. In the next frame, the same two nerve cells, post-Zoloft: neurotransmitters every which way. Fiesta!

Psychoanalysis was out, and psychopharmacology was in. During the 1990s, psychiatrists and ordinary people alike learned to think of a wide variety of mental problems as chemical imbalances, and came to see chemical-balancing medications as the most sensible response. The shift transformed the practice of psychiatry, with analytic methods giving way to a focus on the pharmaceutical management of symptoms that was, indeed, more reminiscent of general medicine than of traditional psychiatry. As if to illustrate just how much things have changed in the couple of generations since the golden age of psychoanalysis, a psychiatrist named Daniel Carlat published a three-page think piece in the *New York Times Magazine* in April 2010, in which he described arriving at a novel idea in his practice: he was going to spend a bit of time during each appointment asking his patients what was going on in their lives, and listening to what they had to say.[39]

THE PHRASE "chemical imbalance" sounds great. It conveys a sense of crisp scientific certainty, the promise of detailed technical knowledge about what depression really is. But despite the phrase's appeal, and its ubiquity, the impression that it gives of open-and-shut understanding is misleading. A scientific model is only as good as how well it accounts for facts, and by that measure, our biomedical model of depression is neither fully complete nor unassailable.

We do know that antidepressants increase the availability of neurotransmitters in the brain. And we know that antidepressants make people with depression feel better (though recent research on the placebo effect shows that these effects might not be as robust as we once believed, particularly for people with "mild" or "moderate" depression[40]). But there are still some data that the serotonin-deficiency model of depression can't account for. For example, studies have shown that only about 25 percent of patients with depression actually have lower than average levels of norepinephrine or serotonin.[41] Befuddlingly, while drugs that enhance the availability of serotonin in the brain seem to help alleviate depression, at least one drug that *depletes* brain serotonin has also been found to be an antidepressant—tianeptine, the world's only selective serotonin reuptake enhancer, is on the market in Europe under the brand name Stablon.[42] Some scientists believe that the fact that SSRIs often take several weeks to start working could be a sign that the changes they cause to serotonin levels, which occur within hours of the first dose, trigger other, deeper changes that are actually responsible for the drugs' antidepressant effect.

While it seems only reasonable to assume that depression, like every other mental state, has a neural substrate, it would be wrong to assume that science has figured out just what this substrate is, or discovered parameters that allow us to distinguish between pathological and nonpathological feelings. Antidepressants have been shown to improve the moods of people with DSM-diagnosable depression, as well as of people who are merely sad.[43] As several psychiatrists pointed out to me, there is no physical test for depression or any other mental disorder. Many clinicians hope and trust that there will be such a test someday—but given that mood is a continuum, the precise spot where "normal" becomes "disordered" will have to be agreed upon, as an act of human judgment. The phrase "chemical imbalance" gestures at the truth, while deftly concealing all that we don't know, as well as the quotient of subjective reasoning that plays a part in any discussion of mental disorder.

The biomedical model of depression is often spoken about as a challenge to earlier models—as if the illness could be "psychological" or "biological," but not both. In fact, these interpretations don't need to be mutually exclusive. The idea that depression is caused by an excessive reaction to the loss of an important relationship and the idea that depression constitutes a malfunction of the serotonin system in the brain could describe two ways of approaching the same phenomenon. It seems only reasonable to assume that our states of mind arise from an interaction of our individual biological tendencies with our life experiences, just as our physical health is the result of a mysterious conversation between our genetic makeup and the treatment we subject our bodies to each day. But instead of expanding on, enriching, and complicating existing knowledge about psychology, our burgeoning understanding of neuroscience has tended to sweep older approaches aside. (Trying to get at this same sense of overcorrection within his discipline, the eminent psychiatrist Leon Eisenberg famously observed near the end of his long career that while psychiatry in the first half of the twentieth century had been virtually "brainless," psychiatry near the end of the twentieth century had grown virtually "mindless.")

In fact, some of the most interesting neuroscience research of the last fifteen years does seek to explore the interface of lived experience and biological reality. Work on "gene-environment interactions" examines the complex interrelationships between the environments we live in and the brains that filter them. Researchers like Bruce McEwen of Rockefeller University in New York City have begun to illuminate how environmental factors such as chronic stress can impact the brain (he has found, for example, that just a few weeks of stress can shrink the volume of the brain's hippocampus, and that a single stressful event can perceptibly change the amygdala), and how both brain-based and environment-based intervention can mitigate them. Such work has led some clinicians to speak of a "biopsychosocial" model of mental disorder, one that appreciates the interrelated contributions of genetic, psychological, and environmental forces. But such blended models face an uphill battle on the road to influence: chemical imbalance is easier to grasp, and pharmaceutical approaches are simpler to implement—and to market—than environmental ones.

While DSM doesn't formally espouse the biomedical model of depression, it is frequently associated with it. In their book *The Loss of Sadness*, Allan Horwitz and Jerome Wakefield, a sociologist and a social work professor, explore the profound effect that the DSM definition of depression has had on the way that we approach emotional problems. They point out two features that make this definition unique. Most cultures, they write, have recognized a state of sadness so protracted and pronounced that it is best considered not a mere feeling, but an affliction. In most times and places these states have been defined with reference to context: sadness becomes pathological when it is grossly out of proportion with what a situation warrants. Our own society's definition of disorder was contextual until not long ago. In DSM-II, for example, depressive neurosis is described as an "excessive" reaction of depression; part of the diagnosis was the clinician's comparison of the patient's symptoms with what was going on in the patient's life. But in DSM-III, not only is the doctor not required to take into account what is happening in the patient's life, but he's also not supposed to.

The second unique feature of the DSM definition of depression, they write, is that DSM attempts to make depression into an absolute category. Many historical models of depression posited not a binary distinction between sick and well, but a long continuum between melancholy illness and complete health. The ancient Greeks, from whom we get our oldest descriptions of depressive illness, had such a system. They defined melancholic illness as an excess of black bile, one of the four bodily substances or "humors" that were thought to be responsible for illness and ordinary temperament alike. People with a melancholic disposition were moody and self-deprecating, but as long as these traits didn't get out of hand, the people who had them weren't considered to be ill. Pathological sadness wasn't different from ordinary sadness in kind, only in degree. But the modern DSM doesn't deal in shades of gray. It was designed to create clarity, filtering out people who do have a disorder from those who don't.

It is an understandable desire. And yet, Horwitz and Wakefield argue that in striving for clarity and consistency, the modern DSM has thrown out clinical accuracy to a worrying degree. They claim that there are any number of life events, like a romantic breakup or the loss of one's job, that could cause a person to meet the DSM criteria for major depression for two weeks or more. Such people are not suffering from a mental disorder, but DSM's lack of attention to context means that they are often erroneously classified as cases of depression. (The two-week cutoff for diagnosing a major depressive episode itself appears to be arbitrary, born more from a wish for standardization than from any scientific principle. An earlier document from which the DSM-III team drew heavily for its work placed the diagnostic cutoff for depression at one month instead.) This doesn't mean that people who are feeling very sad don't want or need aid, only that a depression diagnosis might not be the most accurate or helpful response.

All in all, Horwitz and Wakefield conclude that the modern DSM is incapable of distinguishing between ordinary and disordered sadness. As such, they say, it has greatly expanded the number of people who are seen as having depressive illness—and the number of people who are treated with antidepressants. Recently they've had a glint of agreement from an unlikely source: Robert Spitzer, the psychiatrist in charge of the committee that wrote DSM-III, who once claimed that the new manual was meant to be "a defense of the medical model as applied to psychiatric problems,"[44] went on the record on a BBC documentary in 2007 admitting that he too saw a problem in the DSM's decontextualized approach:

SPITZER: "What happened is that we made estimates of prevalence of mental disorders totally descriptively, without considering that many of these conditions might be normal reactions, which are not really disorders. That's the problem. We were not looking at the context in which those conditions developed."

INTERVIEWER: "So you have effectively medicalized much of ordinary human sadness, fear—ordinary experiences, you've medicalized them."

SPITZER: "I think we have, to some extent."[45]

But never mind the problems, or the simplifications. Every age has placed its spin on depression's mystery. The Greeks used the idea of the four humors; people in the Middle Ages described melancholy as a loss of faith in God's love; Freud saw Oedipal conflict at the heart of everything. And almost within my lifetime, my society has come up with its own explanation—neither more nor less implausible, in its own way, than any of these earlier ones. Chemical imbalance is a powerful metaphor. It is easy to understand. There's something that can even seem intuitive about it. (Discussing his own antidepressant use in *Newsweek* in 1997, the novelist Walter Kirn wrote that after years on medication, he had started to visualize his own serotonin levels moving up and down "according to the weather, the time of year, and what I've had for lunch."[46]) The serotonin idea has the appeal of a totalizing theory, a simple explanation for something complex. It assails us at once with the authority of science and with the ease of something you imagine you can almost feel yourself.

To have a mood disorder in the 1990s meant grappling with the idea of having a real biological disease. Where somebody in the 1960s would have been prompted by the dogmas of the day to pick over their life history and look for deep inner conflicts or subconscious losses, people in our time had to encounter the idea of what it meant to have a malfunctioning brain. And that shift made a difference, not just in terms of which medications people took but also in terms of the way they understood themselves and their experiences. Chemical imbalance wasn't just a theory; it was a story that all of us who took antidepressants had to hold up against our own life story, to fit into it somehow or to consciously reject.

3 | STARTING OUT

During the first few months after I started taking Zoloft, I kept catching myself thinking back to my childhood. I was replaying my earliest memories and, I realized, trying to distill from them some image of the kind of kid I'd been.

It was hard to picture myself from the outside, but when I tried I saw a child who was dreamy, thoughtful, and often worried. I remembered feeling confident and happy at home. My mother told me I'd been bossy and lively as a toddler, a diminutive, redheaded autocrat, and I could believe her. Outside of the house, I hadn't felt nearly so sure of myself. A lot of my early memories seemed tinged with fear, or just an all-purpose eeriness. I remembered wanting to feel connected to the other kids in preschool and kindergarten, but not always knowing how. They seemed so carefree, so thoughtless, so loud. Sometimes I forgot myself and blended with them. But at other times, the feeling that my dad called anxiety would descend for days or weeks, and nothing would feel right. That feeling clenched my stomach, pinched my breath, kept me awake in the dark while the red glowing numbers of the digital clock marched on and on toward morning.

It had been a while since I'd returned to these memories.

But the idea of being a depressed person brought them back from deep storage; it seemed to demand that I reevaluate the past in light of the present, searching for patterns. If what I'd just been through was depression, then what about those times back then? Seen from this new perspective, they seemed like evidence toward the conclusion that Sam had been right—that there really *was* something wrong with me, and that I had always been this way.

Medical anthropologists speak of something called "illness identity," the sense of oneself as sick that parallels the actual experience of being unwell. Without meaning to, I was combing back over my life and revising it into a slightly new story, one that incorporated the idea of my being at least a little bit afflicted. I found that not only was this kind of editing not hard to do, but it was also almost irresistible.

Taking antidepressants is a complicated activity because it takes place on at least two levels. There's the literal level of feelings and actions: we suffer; we see doctors; we receive treatment and feel better, or don't. But there is also an invisible level on which we assign meaning to these experiences. We develop theories about why we felt bad in the first place, why we have chosen the treatments we did, and why they help. Along the way we subtly adjust our self-understanding to incorporate what we've been through.

David Karp is a sociologist who has pointed out that in every experience of depression and treatment, the patient moves through a series of predictable stages—from a vague sense that something is wrong; through a crisis; to the recognition that he has a real problem that must be defined, explained, and managed. Each stage, says Karp, invites revisions to one's sense of self.[1] Talking to people about their own antidepressant stories made me appreciate the simple brilliance of Karp's idea. Dividing the experience into steps allows us both to see what every antidepressant experience has in common and appreciate the variety that is possible at every turn. In this chapter I'll use a collection of my interviewees' voices to talk about how other people got started on antidepressants and began to modify their own identities in response.

WHEN I BEGAN to conduct interviews for this book, I realized I was far from the only antidepressant user who described feeling different from a young age. Christine was in her mid-thirties when we spoke. She had grown up in Denmark, attended graduate school in the United States, and returned to Europe to live before her children were born. I reached her one afternoon on a grainy video-Skype connection that revealed, with a transatlantic time lag, a pretty woman with dark hair, whose slight Scandinavian accent only seemed to make her speech more expressive.

"I've been battling with anxiety my whole life," she told me, "all the way through childhood." Christine felt that her difference was both rewarding and troubling.

> I was very emotional, and sensitive I guess, to everything.
> To life in general. More sensitive than other kids. I always
> pictured myself as this person in black and white, who was
> almost see-through. Everyone else was like colorful and
> alive, and I was just this black-and-white, fragile person. But
> I could feel everything; I could feel everyone around me, all
> their ups and downs.   —*Christine, age thirty-six*

Others expressed a similar idea:

Some of my earliest memories are of being afraid of things. With a lot of fear and anxiety around what I would think are pretty common activities for a child. And all I really knew was that my mom was frustrated with it and that other kids around me didn't understand it; I got teased a lot about being afraid and being sad. —*Ben, age thirty-nine*

My entire life I was always kind of the shy one. I wasn't very social, and that's just kind of the person that I've always been. And as I got into high school, I tried to push myself out of that comfort zone, and tried to be social, but it was still very difficult for me. So I was awkward, and I did outrageous things to get attention, like I colored my hair pink. I started getting the rep for being the weird person, and that never bothered me. —*Shannon, age twenty-six*

Many of those who described a sense of apprehension, difference, or awkwardness in childhood referred to their feelings as an "it." They were aware of these feelings but didn't yet conceive of them as a specific problem. "I know when I was forced to give it a name, when I felt like I had to contend with it as something 'other,'" wrote Anne, a twenty-five-year-old, looking back on the experiences that had led her to start using antidepressants five years earlier. "But if I get to reflecting, then it starts to seem like there isn't really a starting point. Like my life has always been informed by the presence of melancholy and anxiety, and only the intensity has changed." In other people's stories, as in my own, "it" takes on a name and a meaning after a crisis event nudges them into the mental health care system.

Functionally, crisis events are all the same: they mark the point at which someone decides that the problem is serious and requires help. But they come in all shapes and intensities. Some may be recognized as such only in hindsight. Others, like Heather's, are unequivocal.

Heather grew up in a wealthy suburb of Atlanta. Both her parents worked corporate jobs, and Heather and her brothers lived in a comfortable house. Heather is bipolar, with depressions that have been more pronounced than her mania. One afternoon while we sat around her kitchen table in Brooklyn over a snack of crackers and baba ghanoush, she told me the story of her especially spectacular crisis. The year she was fifteen, she explained,

> my brother and I went to ski camp in Italy. And when I was
> there, I was the only girl and there were a million guys, so
> I think that had something to do with it. I was a little bit
> manic, and then when I came home, my mom just sort of
> barked out that this kid in my class was killed in a car ac-
> cident, was run down by a truck, and that just set off this
> horrible reaction of depression. I was beside myself, kind
> of. That was the summer I was fifteen. I started drawing all
> these depressing things and I started writing poetry. Just
> totally withdrawing, and I feel like everything changed
> drastically.

Heather didn't know what was happening to her or even whether the things she was feeling were out of the ordinary, but she did know she was miserable. By fall, she said, "I used to go to a cemetery far away from my house, so I used to walk miles to a cemetery, and I used to sit there, and I used to cut my wrists."

I had my head all shaved, and I shaved off my eyebrows at one point, I just made my mom cry so many times. Or I'd bang my head on a wall. I was like, "I'm *so* miserable, I can't feel anything!" I think that's why people do that to begin with, you're just so numb.

The cutting?

Yeah. Cutting's just like, "Do I feel this? I don't even feel this." And the fact that I can do this to myself is horrifying. And it's also like, "Please fucking help me! This isn't normal behavior." You're not supposed to self-destruct. You're supposed to keep trying to survive, not trying to like kill yourself.

Within a few months, Heather reached a breaking point. "I was totally depressed," she said.

I was just a zombie. And in December, I overdosed on [the anti-anxiety medication] Klonopin. I took them all, and I remember thinking "Okay, I'm going to die now." I remember lying down on my bed. I was like, "I don't really want to die, I'm just so unhappy, I don't want my life to be like this." So I called Poison Control, and I said, "What happens when you take a whole bottle of Klonopin?" And she was like, "You're going to have seizures and heart failure." She said, "Do you want me to call the ambulance?" And I said "No, I can get a ride." So I went downstairs and I asked my mom, like, "Can you take me to the hospital, I just took all my pills."

—*Heather, age thirty-nine*

Heather told me that her crisis seemed to come out of nowhere. "When I was fifteen, bipolar just kind of hit," she said. Other people pegged their crises to a triggering event, like a breakup or a major life transition. Shannon, a brassy former fashion model who grew up in Wisconsin with her sister and mom, was an excellent student but hated the high school environment. She dropped out six months early and spent a couple of years moving around the country with her boyfriend, arriving in Massachusetts when she was nineteen. "It was there that the adult part of my life really hit me," she said. "'I need a job, I have to pay bills,' that sort of thing. He and I had an apartment together, and I was doing temp jobs." She continued:

I decided I needed to do something with my life, so I went to a community college. But I had the same issue I had with high school; it was slow, it was tedious. So after one semester, I decided not to continue. And that's when the depression really started to set in. It began with the reality that I was nothing at that point. I didn't have a career. I didn't have much to live for, so to speak. My relationship with my boyfriend was falling apart, and I was nervous because there was this intense pressure, at least in the city where I went to high school—by the time you were twenty-three, you were married, you had kids, you had a car, you had a house, you were successful, all this kind of stuff, so that pressure was somewhat ingrained in my head, and I just kind of lost it.

I fell into a horrible depression. I was so nervous I couldn't answer the phone. I couldn't even walk outside to get the mail. I was terrified of anything and everything that was outside of the living space that created the comfort zone. I didn't know what to do. I was at the end.

—*Shannon, age twenty-six*

Other times a situation can seem like a crisis precisely *because* there's no identifiable triggering event, and the seemingly illogical nature of the problem is part of what's disturbing about it:

When I was fifteen I was really sad and anxious, and I was tearful a lot, I would cry in school and I couldn't—I would just lie on the floor in my room and I couldn't get up. I did have this kind of generalized anxiety thing, where I would just look at something and a visual something would snap in my brain that would make me feel horribly anxious. Like, it didn't matter, like a tomato in a commercial, it didn't make any sense. And that was horrible, it was like anything could throw me off and it didn't have any sensible story to it.

—*Rachel, age twenty-eight*

But without exception, everyone who talked to me about their crisis described a sense of isolation. Heather felt compelled to "withdraw" from her family and even became alienated from a sense of her own feelings, which were replaced by numbness. Shannon became depressed when she was having trouble finding a way to fit into the world as a productive adult, and in an unfortunately typical piece of irony, being depressed made it even more difficult for her to connect with others. Lindsay suffered partly out of a sense that she couldn't burden anybody else with her suffering. "By the time I was sixteen, I was definitely struggling with some clear depression," she said.

It's kind of a tough year, I think, for anyone; you're a junior in high school, and that's known to be the really hard one. And then my mother was diagnosed with breast cancer, right before Christmas that year. I was spiraling more and more depressed but just keeping it really to myself. I didn't feel that, in spite of my very loving and supportive family, that at that particular moment I could share any of my pain or contribute to the burden that anyone was under, because my mom was so sick.

At one point I started to fantasize about suicide. I had to have a plan. I could make it through my day as it was, but what if it got a tiny bit worse? So I would visualize cutting my wrists and then calling a teacher who I confided in a lot who lived close to me. Visualizing the blood coming out of my wrists was like a release and a hit of something; it kind of perked me up and gave me a bit of strength. At first it was occasional but then I remember picturing this every five minutes or so in class. And that was kind of my coping mechanism, but I totally didn't feel like I could tell anyone that. —*Lindsay, age twenty-six*

One way of thinking about what crises do is to say that they move people to strike out against their isolation by seeking help. For people who have already moved away from home, this usually means reaching a personal breaking point. Shannon remembers arriving at a clear sense that her problems had become more than she could handle alone.

> Six months later, my boyfriend and I ended up splitting up. But it wasn't long after that ended that I came to the personal realization, I need help. I can't do this on my own. Something is wrong with me, and I can't live the rest of my life this way. At the time, I was only nineteen. And I mean, I can't live until I'm seventy like this. I'm not going to make it to seventy. This is awful. So I got help. I found a local counselor, and I started going to counseling.
>
> —*Shannon, age twenty-six*

For people who are still living at home, though, parents usually play a large role in assessing what is wrong and deciding whether to seek help—and what kind it should be.

> When I was young, I was pretty anxious, and then I had like your classic sort of being nudged away by the cool girls in my school. I was thirteen. And then I became basically anorexic because I was like, I can't deal with this. I was in this small environment, and I was totally unhappy. My parents saw me and they were like "Okay, she needs intervention and it needs to be chemical."
>
> —*Alexa, age twenty-three*

Some people remember their parents as benevolent helpers. "When they put me on drugs, I think it was a great decision," said Alexa, "because I really was wasting away, and I went on them and I was a lot better. I gained the weight right back, I made friends, I joined track, and I think I cared a bit more about school." Lindsay dreaded what would happen after she confided her daydreams about suicide to a high school counselor who was obligated to notify her parents. But she remembers their finding out as a good thing. "My parents were really broken up that I was in that much pain and didn't come to them," she said. Having to talk about it was awkward, but fruitful: Lindsay's parents helped her find a therapist and get on Prozac, and they became more involved in her life in a way that Lindsay welcomed. Jamie, eighteen, and her mother, Patricia, both said that coordinating Jamie's care the year that Jamie was a junior in high school brought them some much-needed closeness as mother and daughter.

But a number of people experienced their parents' involvement with more ambivalence. Particularly when it's not the child's idea, the matter of seeking and sticking with treatment can become a point of conflict between parents and offspring, part of the larger power struggle of adolescence. Rachel remembers resenting antidepressants because she felt as if they were being imposed on her:

My mom decided to take me to be seen. The psychiatrist diagnosed me with obsessive-compulsive disorder and some kind of depression and some kind of anxiety disorder. She gave me some medicine, Paxil, Zoloft, Remeron, one at a time. I was resistant at first to taking medicine.

Do you remember why you were resistant?

Because it felt like my mom's idea, and I wanted not to be controlled by her. —*Rachel, age twenty-eight*

Sometimes parents and children disagree not just about the nature of the problem or the best kind of help to get, but even about whether there is a problem at all. Aaron, who is twenty-two, started taking antidepressants when he was twelve. "I've been on and off antidepressants for about ten years," he recounted.

I don't know basically why I was put on it. I just remember one day I was at the mall, and I ran off to do something and then nobody could find me and they flipped out at me, and I reacted, like I threw a fit, and then when we got home I went up to my room and I just kind of stayed there, and my mom came in maybe fifteen, twenty minutes later after I had calmed down, and she said, "We're going to send you to someone to talk about this," and I had no inkling that this was happening. So I started meeting with this guy. I was in seventh grade at the time. And they recommended that I go on Zoloft. —*Aaron, age twenty-two*

Jessica had a similar story. "I started taking antidepressants in fifth grade," she said.

And it really wasn't me that noticed the problem. I think it was my mom, in conjunction with our family doctor. And I think that my mom was concerned because I just wasn't happy. I was way more unhappy than your average unhappy kid should be, I guess. And I mean, nothing traumatic or horribly terrible had happened to me, so she was kind of wondering what else it could be.　　*—Jessica, age twenty-four*

Unlike the people I described at the beginning of this chapter, Aaron and Jessica started taking antidepressants without passing through a crisis stage, at least not one that they were aware of. Their experiences point to one of the main things that makes using antidepressants as a child or a teenager different from using them as an older person, and that is how much weight the opinions of adults carry. At the most basic level, parents are responsible for their children's welfare and are able to tell children what to do. Beyond that, parents' interpretations of what is happening can make an enormous impression on children, who are likely to believe what they're told. Aaron remembers his parents saying to him, "We've noticed you're very sad, you're very moody all the time," and he instinctively agreed: "I was like 'Oh, yeah, I am.'" And Jessica recalls that

> my mother said "I feel like, and the doctor feels like you'd benefit from doing this [taking medication]," and I was like "All right, whatever, you're my mom and my doctor." It was just kind of a no-brainer for me.　　*—Jessica, age twenty-four*

Jessica has doubts about her diagnosis in hindsight. "Looking back on it, I think there may have been other solutions," she said. "I remember feeling very lonely, and I think that was part of it. It may not have been depression as serious as my mom made it out to be. It seems like she might have—not really exaggerated, but my mom has this way of kind of getting her way from the doctor. [If] she feels that I might benefit from a medication, she'll kind of ask him, pointing at this particular idea. She benefits from it; she's actually still on Wellbutrin." Aaron said that while he occasionally second-guesses his parents' choice to put him on medication, "I trust that they probably made the decision they thought was best at the time. I'm glad I was on it, even if I still have that difficult relationship of not knowing whether I want to be on it at any given point."

Friction between parents and children about help-seeking can go both ways, though. I still vividly remember the day I told my friend Joshua that I was going to be working on a book about young people and antidepressants. "I *wish* I'd been put on antidepressants when I was younger," he said fiercely. "Things could have been really different for me." In our culture, adolescents are expected to be moody and to start pulling away and hiding more of their inner lives from their parents, a state of affairs that can leave parents in the dark about how their children are feeling. (I'll also never forget a conversation in which I told my mother that I actually remembered most of high school fondly, as a happy and exciting time. *"What?!"* she almost screamed at me, so surprised was she to hear this. "But you were so . . . horrible!") It can also leave everyone confused about what feelings are to be considered normal. Sometimes this miscommunication can be perceived in hindsight as tragic. Teresa, a twenty-five-year-old in Iowa, wrote to me about finally receiving effective treatment in her twenties for the depression she'd first started to feel at age seven. She described it as "this horrible malaise that would gradually deepen into sleeping *all the time* (seriously, I would come home, go to bed at 4:00 P.M., and wake up at 7:00 A.M. to go back to school. And I'd do this every day)." Teresa always felt that her problems were an illness that needed medical attention. She pushed her parents to get her some help, but with no luck:

> My parents didn't take me to the doctor because (a) they couldn't afford it, and (b) they assumed it was just teenage angst and anxiety, not something "really wrong." They've since told me that they regret it immensely.
>
> —*Teresa, age twenty-five*

Because everyone I interviewed for this book took antidepressants, they all at some point received a diagnosis—for depression, an anxiety disorder, obsessive-compulsive disorder, or one of the hundreds of other conditions in the DSM. Getting a "label" is an important step. Not only does it usher one into the world of pill-taking, but almost by definition, it also has a bearing on one's sense of identity. Nearly everyone I talked to reacted strongly to being diagnosed. But these reactions ran to two polar extremes.

About half of the people I talked to found getting a diagnosis to be an enormous relief. As I discussed in the last chapter, our society over the last thirty years has moved away from seeing many common mental problems as psychological in nature, and toward seeing them as medical—less like facets of personality, and more like diseases that you develop or "catch." These days, diagnosis confronts people with a biomedical explanation for their suffering. Some people specifically told me they took comfort in the biomedical view that came along with their diagnosis.

Thinking of their problems as concrete and physical allowed them to say, at last, "It's not my fault!" They also mentioned the benefits of feeling like they were part of a group, and of finally having an explanation for a set of feelings that had once seemed frighteningly strange.

When I got my diagnosis, I felt absolutely relieved. Finally I wasn't just *crazy*. I had something literally physically wrong with me. And more than that, I had hope that it would go away, or at least get better. —*Teresa, age twenty-five*

To tell you the truth, I think it was probably very comforting. Having depression was kind of saying you belong to a group. I mean, everybody's alone in their sadness, but [to be diagnosed was] to say that you're not necessarily alone-alone in your sadness. At the time, though, I didn't know that there were any other people my age who were having that. But calling it depression was comforting, yes.

—*Abby, age twenty-eight*

I didn't get a proper diagnosis until college. I think I was so relieved actually. And I think it's really because, when you get hit with mental illness, you do not know what you are hit with. And it's the mystery of the illness that is terrifying. With mental illness, there are horrible things happening to you and you don't know what it is, and first getting diagnosed or first getting help is the best thing, because from there on, you're aware that, like—"What is this thing? Let me pick it apart, and let me deal with it." And when you pick it apart, it's not that bad. —*Heather, age thirty-nine*

But an equally large and vociferous group had an almost completely opposite reaction. These people told me that getting a diagnosis made them feel "broken." They focused not on how the diagnosis removed blame, but on how it reified the problem, making it seem big, real, scary, and totally beyond their control. Ben, who developed depression and agoraphobia in high school, said:

In general, I did feel that taking antidepressants was a stigma. To me, I guess it was more evidence that I just wasn't right. That something was fundamentally wrong with me. I already had some feelings along those lines, and this was another example of why. And so taking the medication, while in some senses it was probably a relief, to be given something that was going to help me, I think that by and large the feeling was probably, "Of course, I'm going to have to take this, because this is what people who can't get on in the world take."
—Ben, age thirty-nine

Do you remember what it felt like to get your diagnosis [at age fourteen]?

Yeah. It felt—it was just so sad. I just felt like a freak. I felt weak. I felt ashamed, just, that I needed this, and that even when I was on them I wasn't normal.
—Alexa, age twenty-three

Others reported feeling dehumanized by their diagnosis, as though it meant that other people would no longer take them or their feelings seriously. "The message I got when I was nineteen," said Leah, remembering the time she was hospitalized and diagnosed with bipolar disorder after her first manic break, "was that I was a mood disorder with legs." Elizabeth's story was more prosaic—she started taking antidepressants for panic and depression in middle school, and has been on them since—but she too felt that her "label" marked her and her problem as different in a way that let others keep her at arm's length.

> It was always seen as something wrong with me. And you know, that's not just with my parents, [but also] my teachers and other adults in my life, and other people my age too saw that kind of thing as just "Oh my god, you're broken, and I don't know why."   —*Elizabeth, age twenty-five*

The way people react to their diagnoses has to do with the question of personal agency. People who welcomed a diagnosis felt that the idea of having a "real" disorder was liberating and that it put them in greater control of their lives. Heather mentioned that having a diagnosis gave her a way to fight back against the "mystery" of the disease. And Teresa explained in a note: "In what some may think is an ironic turn, taking medication has made me feel more in control of my life and my body. My brain was literally trying to kill me before, and now it's not." People who had negative feelings about their diagnosis, on the other hand, usually experienced it as a removal of agency, something that would interfere with their ability to be self-sufficient. Elizabeth said that the idea of having a real mental disease was "disempowering, because it makes you feel like there is nothing you can do."

I avoided diagnosing myself as depressed for a really long time, because I wanted to be someone who could fix her own problems. And to me, taking antidepressants just seemed to say "no," I couldn't fix my own problems.

—*Elizabeth, age twenty-five*

Laura, age twenty-three, said, "I wrestle with the fact that I need Zoloft to function. This makes me feel extremely guilty. I think this is the biggest drawback for me—do I have to have a pill in order to operate in this world?"

Personally, I was squarely in the second group. Zoloft did make me feel better, but the *idea* of having depression was like a fish bone that stuck uncomfortably in my throat. There was something ironic at play. As a kid, I'd often felt shy and strange and out of sync with other people. As I got older these feelings had lessened, but they'd never entirely gone away. Getting a diagnosis and beginning to take Zoloft interacted with them interestingly. On the one hand, the medication *did* make me feel more gregarious and relaxed, more unreflectively a part of things, in a way I'd always wanted. But the diagnosis itself worked in the opposite direction. Having a label seemed like official confirmation of my oldest fears: that I really was different, that I didn't belong. In a way, the therapeutic effects of the medicine seemed trumped by the fact of taking them. It didn't matter if I felt better, I thought to myself, in a certain mood; the salient thing was that I needed medication in the first place.

A label also felt like something to hide, a ticklish fact that might cause other people to write me off if they knew about it. A month or two after I started to take Zoloft, I met a tall, laconic freshman named Jeff, who quickly became my much-beloved boyfriend. I eventually told Jeff that I was taking antidepressants, and he seemed okay with it, though it was hard to tell what he really thought—he came from a stoic family of farmers in Texas who didn't *do* depression, let alone take pills for it. My secret out, I lived with the fear that Jeff saw or would come to see me as crazy, and that this would give him good reason to reject me if he wanted to.

FOR MOST OF the people I talked to, medication worked, at least to some degree. A few described their medication experiences as near miraculous. "Going on Prozac was literally going from black and white to color," said Mark. When he first started medication as a law student in his early twenties, he'd felt overwhelmed by depression and anxiety for most of his life. Mark has been on an antidepressant regimen for fifteen years now, but I could still hear the excitement, relief, and even joy in his voice when he remembered first finding effective treatment.

Not everyone has such a powerfully transformative experience, of course. But the majority of people I talked to said they found antidepressants helpful with the problems they started to take them for.

My therapist suggested that I go to a psychiatrist for screening. I'd been trying a lot to bolster my mood by working out more and by, I dunno, thinking about it, and it was rough. So I went and the psychiatrist put me on an SSRI. And it really helped. Within a couple weeks I felt like I was me again, and I hadn't been me for a long time.

—*Claire, age thirty-two*

[Zoloft] helps me not feel despair. I guess that's kind of vague, but when despair actually feels tangible, then there's nothing vague about it, you know.   —*Paul, age twenty-six*

Within a few weeks [of starting Prozac at sixteen], I felt a really big difference. You know, life was still filled with problems. But suddenly it was just, they were problems, not this overbearing force. Right now, I'm taking 40 milligrams of Celexa. I went down to 10 at one point, and it's very interesting to me; it's so clear when things aren't working, within a few days everything is wrong, I'm very anxious. It's been surprising how cut and dried it is.   —*Lindsay, age twenty-six*

I started taking [Lexapro], and within a week, I felt like a human being again. I could feel something changing inside of me. I could feel this different kind of light, this support, this capability that I didn't have before. It was very supportive. It was kind of like someone was holding my hand the entire time.   —*Shannon, age twenty-six*

There's no question that antidepressants help. Before I started taking Lexapro this last time, I couldn't fall asleep or eat unless I was drunk first. I couldn't maintain normal affect long enough to sit through class and had to leave to cry in the bathroom once or more every session. I couldn't interact with my friends normally. I felt like I had absolutely zero control over my actions and my mouth. All of these things got better, within a matter of weeks, once I started taking Lexapro. Everything didn't get wonderful, but it became resoundingly, blessedly okay.   —*Anne, age twenty-five*

A significant minority, however, had mixed or negative reactions. Some people complained about the difficulty of finding the right pill. Because getting started on a drug, giving it time to work, and then tapering down takes weeks or months, finding the right medication can be time-consuming—and, if the side effects are significant, very disruptive. Even people who ended up sticking with medication struggled with side effects. "Each new drug I tried—because I would get immune to them—each one had these terrible side effects," said Alexa. "I got night sweats. I'd wake up, drenched in sweat, and then be cold, so I was basically always sick, which is pretty bad." Certain drugs, notably the SNRI Effexor, cause many people to have hugely uncomfortable symptoms if they miss a dose. "I ran out [of Effexor] over the weekend one time," said Elizabeth, "and that was horrible. You get nightmares that you can't wake up from. You lose the distinction between being awake and asleep." (Effexor, and to some extent Paxil, among other antidepressants, gained notoriety in the 2000s for their ability to cause "discontinuation syndrome"—a pattern of withdrawal symptoms that can last for weeks or months, and may make getting off the drugs difficult.[2])

Others reported just never being sure whether the drugs were having any effect at all.

The psychiatrist gave me some medicine. I don't remember the order, but at one point I was on Paxil, Zoloft, Remeron, one at a time. And everything had side effects that made it not possible to continue. The last med that she put me on was Effexor XR. And that had crazy side effects at first, but there was this encouragement to stay with it. And at that time I was leaving for college. I don't know if the medication really worked or if going to college worked or if I got older, and that worked. I would still get really low and really anxious, and have other symptoms that started in college, but I guess it worked better than the other ones.

—*Rachel, age twenty-eight*

I sometimes hoped that the drugs would do something. Like that as I raised the dose, I'd suddenly start to feel better. I was told that you're supposed to get a very marked reaction the first time it starts to kick in. But I never felt that in a way that could be attributed to the medication, rather than the placebo effect or other things going on in my life. So honestly I was never sure whether they were working.

—*Elizabeth, age twenty-five*

After a crisis, after help-seeking and diagnosis and treatment with medication, after the medication works or doesn't work, and things stabilize again, people begin to integrate their stories and assign meaning to everything that happened. This is the point at which childhoods are revised, where a problem that was once an "it" is solidified into a whole narrative.

A few pages back, I wrote that getting a diagnosis and, especially, taking a medication entail a forceful encounter with a biomedical interpretation of one's suffering. People who encounter this explanation need to accept or reject it as part of their own personal story. Some accept it easily, others do so only with reservations or after the passage of time, and others never quite accept it at all—though if medications work for them, this can lead them to have to do some mental acrobatics: when you find relief from a drug, it's hard to cling to the premise that your problems weren't in some way chemical.

Mark, the former law student, took to a biomedical narrative comfortably and easily. Partly this was because Prozac worked so well for him. Partly it was because the story suggested by Prozac seemed succinctly to explain a lot about his early life. "I'd been, in many respects, as I look back on it, depressed since I was a child, and certainly anxious," Mark told me. But at the time, "I wasn't really that aware of it to say that there was something wrong." He cited one of his earliest memories: "I was two and a half, I guess. Christmas at my father's workplace. It was Santa Claus, and all the little kids were there. And my mother was like, 'You wanna go out?' And I was like, 'Mm-mmm, no!' I was just afraid, to tears, of these people. I was scared to death of it. It was like *Lord of the Flies*." Mark had always known he felt bad. "Depression" was a story that made his early experiences make sense. It snapped his past life into focus, dignified his present, and made him able to believe in a better future. "The idea that depression is a medical illness was just unbelievably empowering, and very important for me," he said. "It took away some of the shame, and gave some hope. And for society, it had a similar effect. It's a potent story that, thankfully, has changed many people's understanding toward people with depression."

Heather, who developed bipolar disorder as a teenager, had never felt depressed in childhood, but she too gravitated toward a chemical explanation for her problem. In fact, she fought for it. (Like Mark, Heather was at the older end of my sample, which might help explain why they both feel so passionate about the medical paradigm. Each mentioned feeling as if they grew up in a climate of awareness where their difficulties either went unrecognized or weren't interpreted correctly.) "The care I got in the 1980s was horrific," said Heather.

> After getting out of the hospital, the individual therapist I had, I went to see her mentor who she had studied under. I saw that woman for six years I think. This is the woman who should have been able to tell what was wrong with me. They were coming up with stuff like, "Oh, your father molested you," all these things, and it was like "No, I'm fucking depressed!"
>
> *They wanted there to be this reason for it.*
>
> I know, and it was chemical. Is chemical.
>
> *—Heather, age thirty-nine.*

Most of the people I talked to accepted the idea of having a real illness more gradually, and with more ambivalence. When antidepressants were first suggested to her in high school, Rachel wrote in an e-mail,

> I was really against [the idea] and quite terrified, but I was backed into a corner by my mother and my psychiatrist, and I hated feeling the way I was feeling and I was in some sense at rock bottom so I didn't care what happened to me. I heard metaphors about bathtubs whose drains suck up water faster than it can come out of the faucet—the water being the serotonin that my brain is not producing fast enough—and I thought they were such bullshit but I was also just too weak and crumpled to really put up enough of a fight.
>
> *—Rachel, age twenty-eight*

But she did start taking medication, and the experience of feeling better on it slowly started to change her views. "Now I feel like a poster child for antidepressants," she said, "because unless I'm in a bad situation, I can function almost as normal. I used to believe that medication was almost never a good idea, but now I believe that there is definitely a place for it." She told me that being on antidepressants had affected her sense of herself in complex ways. After thirteen years on them, she is used to feeling well—that's part of her identity now. At the same time, taking medication for so long has also solidified her sense of having an illness. When I asked Rachel whether she thought that using antidepressants had changed her, she paused and thought. "I don't think that medication has affected me inasmuch as medication shifted my brain chemistry and thus who I am," she said. "But more like I was told that I was depressed and anxious and this and that, and *that* kind of confused me about who I am, more. So that's always there in the background when I think about quitting. Like—maybe I am this crazy person, but the medicine's working."

Other people took medication and found that it helped their symptoms, but they still raged against the conclusion that they were "really" ill. Laura, twenty-three, wrote to me about getting back on Zoloft the previous spring, after she graduated from college. She said the Zoloft was working "very well" but confided that "I hesitated for months about going back on it." Like many people I spoke to, she wanted to resist the feeling that she "needed" a pill, and she fantasized about a future when she might be able to get by without it: "I am still waiting for a moment in my life where everything is a bit more settled, and then perhaps I can get off."

Sometimes a reluctance to settle into the illness identity

suggested by antidepressants led people to try going off their medication. A number of people quit for this reason, only to be rewarded with repeat episodes of depression. Some people became long-term users of antidepressants only after cycling through several such trials and failures. Christine, from Denmark, had a story like that:

> I always had a lot of ups and downs. And that was kind of taken away by Celexa. But the downs were taken away too, and that was helpful. And then every time I stopped, I tried to come off, I fell into a depression, and started back on them again.
>
> *What made you stop to begin with?*
>
> I guess I've never seen myself as really mentally ill, or really depressed. I've never had like a sick period where I've just been lying in bed, I've never had to stay home from school or work or anything. I've never been *crazy*-crazy, I've always been affluent and gone to good schools and held great jobs, and managed a lot of things, I guess. So I thought, why should I be on medication when I'm not crazy? So then I try to stop, but there's this whole falling into a big depression, is not great either. So, it's not good.   —*Christine, age thirty-six*

And I was the same way.

By spring semester of freshman year, I felt well, happy, back to normal. I had great friends, classes were exciting, and I was in love with Jeff. I started to wonder whether I really needed antidepressants anymore. So I decided to test the premise by stopping. There were still things about taking them that bothered me, and quitting seemed like the easiest way of sweeping the whole mess aside.

I didn't tell anyone in the Health Center about my decision. I just tapered down my dosage as I'd read you should. Within a few weeks I was pill free and feeling fine. A little of the anxiety that had departed the semester before returned, but it was nothing I couldn't handle. As people began making their arrangements to return home for the summer, though, I started to wobble. The prospect of saying good-bye to Jeff felt particularly traumatic. We had plans to visit once or twice over the break, and of course there would be next year. But it didn't matter. When I thought about parting even for a little while, I felt a wave of irrational but intense dread. On our last night in town together Jeff and I saw a movie at a local second-run theater and then stopped for pancakes at the Waffle House near the highway. I snuffed back tears all through the meal. Jeff held my hand and said sensible things like "It's only for a summer," while I hated myself for my show of vulnerability.

Back at home in Arlington I tried to pull myself together, but the summer seemed to have gotten off on an awkward footing. I missed my college friends and the structure afforded by classes, papers, and deadlines. My sister was busy with her own friends, and while I saw Sarah and other members of my high school crowd occasionally, it felt as if we were drifting apart. Eventually I landed an internship at the National Museum of Natural History on the Mall in Washington, which I had applied for months earlier. I was to spend six weeks in the arctic anthropology department, taking photographs of a collection of Neolithic stone artifacts that were on loan from a university in Canada. For most of the day, I worked by myself in a cold room filled from floor to vaulted ceiling with taxidermic birds. I had always loved the museum, and it felt amazing to be able to enter my key code each morning and slip through an inconspicuous door tucked behind a fiberglass diorama of a South Sea island, and into a warren of hallways lined with greenish wood shelves stuffed with every manner of specimen—including an alarming number of human skeletons in drawers whose yellowed labels still bore the loops of perfect Victorian penmanship. I took lunch breaks on the steps outside, in the shadow of the big pieces of petrified wood that guard the museum's front entrance. In the gritty summer heat of Washington I watched pigeons peck at pretzel crumbs and listened to the happy-tired-cranky din of families on vacation, but the contrast between that bustle and my cold, silent work environment made me feel even lonelier. Everyone else seemed to be doing something that made sense, I thought, while I felt lost and flailing.

Like it had the summer before, my mood drifted out to sea. I cried in the bathroom of the telemarketing office where I moonlighted for extra money. I cried on the steps of the United States Supreme Court, where I sat one day, killing time before work. I cried in the exquisite marble bathroom of the Arctic Anthropology wing of the National Museum of Natural History. I cried at Cold Spring Harbor Laboratories, in Long Island, New York, where I went to visit Jeff at his fancy summer biochemistry internship. I cried on the gently sloping lawn of the tasteful Cape Cod house on the grounds of the Labs, where James Watson, codiscoverer of the DNA double helix, lived with his wife. Seeing Jeff helped, but only temporarily; I spent the visit dreading the moment I would step into the taxi that would carry me back to the Long Island Railroad station and the rest of my life.

I didn't have any good theories about what had unhinged me, but this time, the words to describe it ("depressed, again") and the action to take were closer at hand. On a sweltering D.C.-area day, I drove out to the "behavioral health clinic" where my mother's HMO provided mental health services. The doctor there sat with me for even less time than Sam had, but it didn't surprise me anymore. I came home with a bottle of fiery orange Wellbutrin.

This was the point at which I became committed to medication. After crashing a second time, it was harder to see what was happening to me as a fluke. I still didn't want to use antidepressants, but I started to grudgingly accept it as preferable to what was beginning to seem like the alternative, and the new pills traveled back to school with me. My mother's HMO managed the prescription for the rest of college, fielding refill requests over their automated phone system, sending giant, geriatric-size bottles of pills from Virginia to Oregon in tough plastic mailers.

On the one hand, it seemed like the evidence was piling up that I did have a chemical imbalance—whatever that really meant. But though I found it ever harder to reject the story about me suggested by medication, I never really accepted it either. Unlike Mark, who saw in his childhood the beginnings of a disease he wanted no part of, and unlike Heather, who saw in her childhood a whole kid that bipolar disorder later obscured, I harbored more personal feelings about my "it." Christine told me that when she was little, she'd felt fragile but also sensitive and perceptive. I had similar mixed feelings about my own young self: she seemed skittish, intense, prone to get lost in thoughts she couldn't explain. But even though I'd hated this difference, I'd also loved it. And for no especially defensible reason except that it was what I believed, I was afraid that antidepressants were going to sweep away those private feelings, spell the end of the strange, mystical kid I'd been.

I never wanted to feel the way I had felt over the summer again, and if antidepressants were the price to pay not to have to, I would take them. But I felt angry that the choice had come to that, and I wasn't quite ready to embrace the idea that what I had was really a sickness. Like Laura, I never stopped cherishing the idea of some future day when I'd be able to live without medication.

Most of the time, though, I dealt with the cognitive dissonance by ignoring it. Taking pills quickly becomes a habit, and there was plenty to distract me. College rolled on, in its demanding and engaging way. Jeff dropped out after our sophomore year and moved back to Texas, to my shock and sadness, but I weathered his leaving. Eventually there were other boyfriends, new friendships, a series of run-down student apartments that all seemed wonderful in their own way. I switched majors, started going to the gym, made Phi Beta Kappa at last. I worked summer jobs and turned myself into a student to contend with. I wore nylon vests, got an old road bike, and started to blend in with the Pacific Northwest. It's not that I never felt bad; some months and semesters were better than others. But I didn't crash again the way I had those two times. And while I never did get to like the idea of taking antidepressants, it often became the sort of habit that you can forget about, in the loud rush of life.

4 | DECADE OF THE BRAIN

The commercial started out just like any other. There was the big house, the sunlit yard, the pretty lady, all in the soft focus of a suburban daydream. You might have assumed it was an ad for—dish soap? Diamonds? Something grown-ups like to have for breakfast? But after a few seconds, you'd have noticed something that was unlike other ads. It was an aura of gloom. Inside the house the lady, a brunette, stood too close to the window. The dim light around her contrasted with the brightness outside, where children played and cheerful voices called out. The woman inclined her head and fingers toward the glass in an attitude of worried longing; she looked like Betty Crocker playing the role of Boo Radley. There was a party going on out there, but she was stuck, indoors, behind this wall of glass. Was it a yeast infection? Then the voice-over came in.

Over light piano music, a woman spoke:

"Doctors define social anxiety disorder as an intense, persistent fear and avoidance of social situations. Has overwhelming anxiety significantly impaired your work or social life? Paxil offers new hope."

In the second half of the commercial, warm gold light had replaced the cold blue tones. The curtains parted. Beyond them, grown-ups with sweaters tied around their shoulders, preppie-style, embraced politely beside tables spread for a garden party. The voice continued, faster now: "Side effects may include decreased appetite, dry mouth, sweating, nausea, constipation, sexual side effects in men and women, yawn, tremor, and sleepiness." Two guys roughhoused with a kid in a football jersey. A man in a dark suit rose to accept a professional award. The piano tinkled a last few poignant notes.

"Will you ask your doctor for more information about Paxil? Do it today. Your life is waiting."[1]

WHILE I WAS trying to get used to the idea of having a chemical imbalance, the culture at large was busy developing a wholesale fascination with SSRIs. Between the early 1990s and the early 2000s, representations of antidepressants in the media abounded. These were the years when it began to seem that you couldn't open a newspaper or magazine, set foot in a bookstore, or turn on the television without being assailed by a laudatory or hand-wringing statement about antidepressants—or a straight-up sales pitch. One reason why SSRIs carried such force as a topic of discussion was that we were ambivalent about them, in the true sense: not indifferent, but simultaneously attracted and repelled. Antidepressants spoke to some of our deepest desires while activating some of our deepest fears; they appealed to certain cherished cultural values while threatening to violate others.

And it was our collective inability to come down conclusively on one side or the other that helped keep Prozac* in the spotlight almost continuously. The two-minded attitudes about antidepressants that we forged during the SSRIs' first decade persist to this day. Because the tensions that made antidepressants interesting then still inform the way people think and talk about their own medication use, it's worth taking a closer look at what those tensions are and how they came to be.

THE COMMERCIAL AND cultural antidepressant bonanza got off to a good start in the year 1990, when President George H. W. Bush issued a proclamation naming the 1990s the "Decade of the Brain." He called upon Americans "to observe that decade with appropriate programs, ceremonies, and activities."[2] Two of those activities, whether he intended it or not, included acquiring a taste for Prozac and cultivating a new, particularly 1990s-inflected awareness of mental illness. Though Americans had always had their psychological complaints—remember the crazes for Miltown and Valium—during the 1990s those problems were translated out of the thorny psychoanalytic language of previous decades and into the bland, biomedical terminology of the DSM. Under the influence of that new vocabulary, the 1990s saw what Carina Chocano, writing for *Salon*, called "sudden syndrome proliferation syndrome."[3] It seemed like every day, some strangely named ailment that appeared to describe familiar behavior in new terms—social anxiety disorder, premenstrual dysphoric disorder, seasonal affective disorder—was

---

*From here on, in keeping with tradition, I will use "Prozac" to refer to the whole class of SSRIs, unless it's clear I am talking about Prozac specifically.

turning out to be biological in nature and treatable with medication.

How did it happen? Almost from the start, the SSRIs seemed uniquely able to capture the public's imagination. They were the center of a highly appealing story of scientific progress: a new, magic-bullet solution for a once-intractable problem. Prozac made the cover of *Time* magazine twice during the 1990s. In 1992, in a cover package introducing many Americans for the first time to the idea of chemical treatments for mental illness, *Time* considered questions like "Is Freud Finished?," noting that "with the advent of new drug therapies, Freudian analysis has become almost irrelevant to the treatment of severe depression and schizophrenia."[4] Neuroscientists, the articles explained, were enjoying the bounty of "a burst of new ideas about how the mind works," including the idea that many mental disorders "are at their core disruptions of normal brain chemistry and can often be treated as such."[5] Readers were told of practical solutions for the treatment of depression, which was now presented as being both common (like depressive neurosis), and biological in origin (like endogenous depression), as if these two older categories had been merged into one new one. "It is the treatment of ordinary depression—the crushing despondency that strikes more than twelve million Americans each year," the *Time* article continued, "that represents mental health's greatest success story." Thanks to "a crop of new, highly specific antidepressant drugs," treatment of depression was becoming fast and easy: "Today depression can be treated—quickly and effectively—in seven cases out of ten. If a second round of treatment is required, the cure rate jumps to 90 percent."[6]

Before long, presidential proclamations and breathless coverage in the press were joined by another stream of media that had great power to make antidepressants visible and shape the way that people thought about them—and about depression itself. In August 1997, the FDA changed a regulation that had prevented drug companies from advertising prescription drugs to the public.* These companies had long been allowed to promote their products to doctors through advertisements in medical journals, and by sending company reps, or "detailers," to doctors' offices to deliver free samples, pens, note cubes, and information about the benefits of particular products. But direct-to-consumer advertising opened up a whole new world.

Soon after that decision in 1997, television commercials for prescription-only drugs became a commonplace. Many people found them funny, and they were, for their strange juxtaposition of typically cheesy advertising images with frank and highly unsexy language about conditions and side effects. (When was the last time you'd heard the word *sweating* in a commercial for anything, antiperspirant included?) Some of the ailments for which treatments were advertised themselves sounded outlandish: thanks to prescription drug advertising, millions of TV viewers had the chance to raise an eyebrow at the idea of a condition called "restless leg syndrome." The mandated side-effect list readouts, too, often veered into bizarre territory: "Tell your doctor if you experience new or increased gambling urges, increased sexual urges, or other intense urges while taking rasagiline."[7]

Funny or not, direct-to-consumer (DTC) ads worked. Certainly the pharmaceutical industry found them worth investing

---

*Currently the United States and New Zealand are the only two developed countries that allow direct-to-consumer advertising of prescription drugs.

in. The amount it allocated for ads to consumers quadrupled between 1997 and 2004, to $4.35 billion.[8, 9] In 2000, every dollar the pharmaceutical industry spent on DTC advertising translated into an additional $4.20 in sales, about four times higher than the rate of return on promotion directly to doctors.[10] The ads changed consumer behavior as well. A 2003 report found that a third of adults had talked to their doctors about a particular medication they had seen advertised. Four out of five who did ended up receiving a prescription, either for the drug they'd asked about or for another drug.[11]

Along with proton pump inhibitors for stomach problems, cholesterol-lowering drugs, and pain medications, antidepressants were one of the classes of pharmaceuticals most heavily promoted under the new regulations. When the Paxil commercial I described at the beginning of this chapter aired in 2000, *Advertising Age* noted that it was "the first sixty-second branded spot ever for a central nervous system drug" on television.[12] Campaigns for the three most popular antidepressants of the time, Prozac, Paxil, and Zoloft, had already appeared in national magazines. In the early 2000s, media consumers became familiar with messages urging them to consider whether sadness, low energy, and loss of interest might be signs of depression, generalized anxiety disorder, or one of the handful of other conditions that SSRIs had been approved to treat, and to "ask their doctor" whether a particular antidepressant might be right for them.

WHILE THE MASS media gushed about the promise of SSRIs in the editorial sections and tried to sell them to us in the advertorial ones, references to Prozac, generally of a more ambiguous nature, abounded in popular culture. In Douglas Coupland's book *Generation X*, which came out in 1991 and introduced a lot of people (including a young-teenaged me) to the myth of the slacker, a character explains, "I was an impostor, and in the end my situation got so bad that I finally had my Mid-twenties Breakdown. That's when things got pharmaceutical."[13] Tank Girl, the brawling, cursing, hedonist heroine of the British comic book series, terrorized the landscape of post-apocalypse Australia, wearing a necklace made of silver-dipped Prozac pills in her eponymous 1995 American movie. (What did it mean? We didn't know, but it seemed bad-ass.) The following year, Homer Simpson cooked up a batch of "homemade Prozac" in his kitchen in Springfield; the panacea seemed to consist largely of ice cream.[14]

Probably the best-known appearance of SSRIs in art during the period occurred in HBO's *The Sopranos*, which first aired in 1999. The show's well-known premise is that its protagonist, Tony Soprano, is the don of New Jersey. He's also a family man, with problems at work and at home, and he's experiencing panic attacks. Tony's somewhat reluctant decision to see a psychiatrist is the catalyst that sets the whole show in motion. In the first episode his new shrink, Dr. Melfi, slides a prescription for Prozac across her stylish glass table. "With today's pharmacology," she tells him, "nobody needs to suffer with feelings of exhaustion and depression."[15] Subsequent episodes track Tony's crime career, his family life, and his progress and lack thereof with medication and talk therapy.

While early trailers for the show mined Tony's medication use for yuks—look at the tough guy on Prozac!—the show quickly settled into its own kind of realism. The fact that Tony took medication was a tip-off about how widespread antidepressants had become: if he could be using them, anyone could. (Besides depicting a changing reality, *The Sopranos* also helped to shape it. In the Canadian magazine *The Walrus*, Wendy Dennis wrote that "as a result of Tony's twice-weekly appointments, many therapists have reported an increase in male patients."[16])As the seasons rolled on, the show took Tony's therapy, pharmaco- and otherwise, as an opportunity to ask serious questions. There is a tension throughout the series between Tony's activities in therapy and his crime career and personal life. Will Prozac make Tony (and by analogy, the rest of us) a better person, or will it just make him *feel* better while he goes on lying and cheating and breaking kneecaps? *The Sopranos* picked up on the fact that Prozac plucked at a very old philosophical conversation about the relationship of being happy to being good.

Some of the depictions of antidepressants in the culture were critical or at least skeptical. It was easy to portray Prozac-taking as a habit of poor little rich folks, something people did to stave off the ennui of not living fuller or more meaningful lives. The 1995 Blur album *The Great Escape* explores the theme of alienation in an affluent, consumerist world. Its song "Country House," which hit number one on the UK charts, paints a portrait of a successful man who moves to the country to escape the pressures of the "rat race." Once there, he indulges heavily in therapeutic culture, "reading Balzac, [and] knocking back Prozac" in an all-out search for equanimity.[17] But the joke is on the man, whose strenuous efforts ("he doesn't drink smoke laugh, takes herbal baths") seem to lead nowhere at all. The end of the song leaves him as self-absorbed and fundamentally dissatisfied as it found him.

"Country House" partakes of the same tradition as the Rolling Stones' "Mother's Little Helper," a song about tranquilizers that appeared exactly thirty years before it. The Stones' protagonist is a busy woman who feels overworked and underappreciated, and reaches for pharmaceuticals to ease the strain. ("And though she's not really ill, there's a little yellow pill/ She goes running for the shelter of a mother's little helper."[18]) In both songs, whatever relief our characters find seems like false consciousness: the pills provide a veneer of calm that only masks larger problems. And those problems, it's implied, are social or existential, not medical. We suspect that the man in the country house is actually suffering from his own navel-gazing disengagement from life, and the housewife, perhaps, with mortality itself, if we take the tip-off in the song's opening words: "What a drag it is getting old." Both songs exemplify what I call the romantic critique of psychopharmaceuticals, a view that entails the idea that popping a pill can be a way of turning one's back on life, numbing psychic pain rather than confronting its real causes.

The romantic critique of antidepressants returns over and over again in art and music. It appears in *Garden State*, the 2004 film in which the protagonist, Andrew, a twentysomething man played by Zach Braff, uses the occasion of a trip home to New Jersey to go off the battery of antidepressants and mood stabilizers that his psychiatrist father has had him taking for years. He reconnects with old friends and forms a relationship with a quirky young woman played by Natalie Portman, connections that are vivifying where his medications merely numbed and stifled him. As the film progresses, Andrew loosens up, finally beginning to smile and laugh. See, the movie says, he doesn't need pills! He needs *love*! He needs to *feel*! He needs Natalie Portman! The love-conquers-all plot builds up toward a cleansing rainstorm and a literal primal scream at the bottom of a quarry.[19]

The romantic critique is easy to grasp and smugly satisfying, but it's also a little sophomoric. It portrays recovery as being as easy as being willing to look your problems in the eye, a proposition that most serious chroniclers of depression and anxiety have understood just isn't true. David Foster Wallace gives depression a more nuanced and disquieting treatment in his short story "The Depressed Person," whose protagonist suffers terribly even as she uses her depression to manipulate others and excuse gross acts of selfishness. Though the story doesn't mention antidepressants directly, it reads like a scathing indictment of the idea that getting better is as simple as wanting to.

PROZAC CAPTURED THE popular press and made its way into art, but Peter Kramer might have been its first philosopher. His 1993 book *Listening to Prozac* deserves special mention because it did so much to set the terms of the debate about the SSRIs; the conversations that we still have today about how antidepressants affect the self originated with Kramer's descriptions of what the drugs do. The book became a phenomenon of its own, climbing into the *New York Times* bestseller list and sticking.

In the book Kramer, who is a psychiatrist in Providence, Rhode Island, describes prescribing the then-new drug Prozac to his patients. He argues that Prozac is unlike any drug he had prescribed before. Not only is it more powerful, but it also appears to be more global, changing his patients' very personalities. He sketches for us the "rough around the edges" architect who loses his depression but also, unaccountably, his taste for pornography; the administrator who after a lifetime as a shy, self-effacing person becomes assertive and vivacious. Prozac, Kramer concludes—and rightly or wrongly, this has become part of our collective consciousness about SSRIs—goes way beyond the previous antidepressants and subtly alters the self itself.

Listening to Prozac is a book fueled by ambivalence. Prozac thrills Kramer the clinician: he portrays the drug as stupendously effective. But it unsettles Kramer the humanist profoundly. He believes that the pill fosters biological reductionism, revealing as chemical what Kramer and his patients alike had once considered psychological. "When one pill at breakfast makes you a new person," Kramer writes, "it is difficult to resist the suggestion, the visceral certainty, that who people are is largely biologically determined."[20] And that thought seems to Kramer to cut against the notions of free will, personal responsibility, and the importance of trying hard, on which we've built our democratic society.

Kramer believes that Prozac has a way of instructing people about what's pathological and what isn't; that's what is meant by the title of the book. Every quirk that yields to the drug's effects is cast in a new light of suspicion: was it really a symptom of disorder all along? Kramer's once-shy patient, Tess, eventually discontinues Prozac, but she returns to Kramer's office some months later, complaining that she is "slipping"; she tells her doctor simply that without Prozac, "I am not myself." Kramer is floored. "After all," he writes, "Tess had existed in one mental state for twenty or thirty years; she then briefly felt different on medication. Now that the old mental state was threatening to re-emerge—the one she had experienced almost all her adult life—her response was 'I am not myself.' But who had she been all those years if not herself?"[21] Kramer feels uneasy as he contemplates writing out a prescription for a person who in no way satisfies the definition he'd worked with all his adult professional life of any mental illness. He feels he is medicating not a disease but a personality. But Tess wants the Prozac, and he can't see what harm it will do, so he reaches for his pad.

Kramer's book is portentous but prescient. It both foresees and, in the way it sets up the debate, *creates* the future of our discourse about the SSRIs. The cover of the book features a graphic that I remember finding terrifying when I was in ninth grade and first saw a copy lying around my parents' house. A figure of indeterminate gender, drawn in runny pastel, is lifting off his/her own face as though it were a mask—pulling it straight off the top of his/her own head like the burned outer layer of a marshmallow toasted over a campfire. Underneath there is no face at all, just a streaming void of flesh tones. Kramer was afraid that Prozac would obliterate the self as we knew it—that it would usher in an age where all the features of our personalities, instead of being given and fixed, would become optional. ("Since you only live once, why not do it as a blonde? Why not as a peppy blonde?"[22]) He coined the phrase "cosmetic psychopharmacology"[23] for this hypothetical state of affairs, and though he couldn't put his finger on how he could object to the practice on ethical grounds, it nevertheless filled him with unease. It seemed to threaten the whole enterprise of psychiatry, which was, at least when Kramer had done his training, about finding meaning in suffering and making deliberate, incremental change. Prozac, he fretted, might even overturn the "continuous, autobiographical human self," which had been psychiatry's one true subject.[24]

The appeal of cosmetic psychopharmacology is obvious. Who among the striving, white-collar people who read the book wouldn't identify the usefulness of a substance that caused a state not of intoxication but of hypereffectiveness: increased energy, reduced social friction? Kramer described a drug that could make you more relaxed in your dealings with others, warmer, more focused on business and pleasure alike. Kramer may have been iffy about his subject, but his best-selling book was probably one of the best pieces of promotion that the drug could possibly get. It's hard to imagine that *Listening to Prozac* didn't inspire a lot of people to have a chat with their doctors about whether an SSRI was right for them.

And yet Kramer wasn't the only one who found the notion of a world where every aspect of our personalities is up for revision unsettling. If there was something about the pill Kramer described that inspired desire in us, there was also something that stimulated fear. Feeling "better than well," as Kramer called the state that Prozac could induce in some, sounded tantalizing on the one hand, but uncanny and maybe even repellent on the other.

There's a *New Yorker* cartoon from around this time that I like because its humor hangs on both of these reactions. It's a three-frame strip titled "If They Had Prozac in the 19th Century." Each frame is an oil-pastel portrait of a heavyweight thinker, looking happy and saying something inane. Karl Marx is smiling; he looks like Santa Claus. "Sure!" he's exclaiming. "Capitalism can work out its kinks!"[25] The cartoon is funny because it zeroes in, absurdly, on our hopes and fears about Prozac. Marx just seems so cheerful. Who wouldn't want to be cheerful like that? And yet if Marx had been happier in a gee-whiz kind of way, he wouldn't have been the Marx we know. There'd have been no *Communist Manifesto*; history might have run a different course. Would this have been better for Karl Marx? For the rest of the world? The awkwardness of not knowing, the absurdity of weighing something like Marx's intellectual legacy against something like the idea of perkiness, is what produces the laugh. This was the dilemma of cosmetic psychopharmacology: we wanted to be happy but we worried that maybe there was something even more important than happiness that we'd unwisely be giving up in the bargain.

THE UNEASY PROSPECT raised by *Listening to Prozac*, of a world chemically purged of shyness, orneriness, and roughness-around-the-edges, helps to explain one notable feature of our national conversation about antidepressants. It is in light of the fears awakened by the idea of cosmetic psychopharmacology and the objections inherent in the romantic critique of antidepressants that we can best understand the claim, used so often in antidepressant advertisements and by psychiatrists and biologically oriented mental health advocacy groups from the 1990s on, that depression is a "real" disease with physical causes. In chapter 2, I talked about the rise of the biomedical model of depression. That rise occurred for a variety of reasons, ranging from the discovery of antidepressants themselves to the psychiatric profession's determination to break out of its humanistic mind-set and become more like the rest of medicine. But the biomedical model of depression also caught on because it was a useful rhetorical tool for selling antidepressants to a public that was wary about taking pills that might change the self, or constitute a mere palliative against the sorrows of everyday life.

Aside from the question of its correctness or incorrectness, the biomedical model of depression was a good way of countering those fears. Accordingly, ad campaigns and other promotional statements for antidepressants have consistently constructed depression—and the other conditions that antidepressants are prescribed for—as true diseases, a logic that paints antidepressants as real medicines, not all-purpose mood brighteners or, as Nathan Kline once described Marsilid, "psychic energizers." If depression is truly an illness, after all, then antidepressants can't be accused of being the chemical equivalent of rhinoplasty.

The claim that depression is a bona fide disease has been promoted almost as heavily over the years as antidepressants themselves. For example, the first direct-to-consumer ad campaign for Prozac, which appeared in *Time* magazine in 1997, is at pains to educate its readers about depression's status as a real disease of physical origin. Under a cartoonish drawing of a thundercloud and the headline "Depression Hurts," informative text describes depression as a medical condition. "Depression isn't just feeling down," the copy reads. "It's a real illness with real causes"—namely, the levels of serotonin in the body, which Prozac can help bring back to normal.[26]

Often, the claim that depression is a real disease is made more specific by likening it to a specific condition, most frequently diabetes. Examples of this comparison crop up everywhere. In the instruction manual for a major, National Institute of Mental Health (NIMH)–funded clinical study of antidepressants, physicians involved in the research were instructed to make sure that their patients "understand that depression is a disease, like diabetes or high blood pressure, and has not been caused by something the patient has or has not done."[27] Several people I interviewed about their own antidepressant use mentioned that doctors had used the diabetes metaphor to explain antidepressants to them at the beginning. Rachel said that when she was in high school and feeling reluctant to start antidepressants, "I heard metaphors from my psychiatrist and my mother about diabetes and how you have to treat that, and that what I was going through was no different." When you start to listen, you hear the claim that "depression is a disease just like diabetes" over and over again—in educational materials, op-eds, and quotes from psychiatrists in newspaper and magazine stories.

Likening depression to diabetes sets up a direct analogy between antidepressants and insulin treatments. It portrays depression as a condition in which the body doesn't make enough of a substance it's supposed to have in abundance—serotonin is to insulin—and, by extension, casts antidepressants as a medically necessary treatment to address that lack. (The comparison also subtly hints that antidepressant use should be chronic and ongoing, as insulin therapy is. Like diabetes, it imagines depression as a permanent condition: something you manage, but not something you really get better from.)

Proponents of the depression-is-a-disease-like-diabetes view argue that their position is important not only because it's correct, but also because it helps to undo a long-standing stigma that has been attached to depression. People with depression, the argument goes, have often been made to feel guilty and weak for not being able to "snap themselves out of it." In contrast to damaging views from the past, which held depression to be a sin, a moral failing, or a character flaw, the biomedical model portrays depression as both real (it's not something you can shake off or will yourself out of) and nobody's fault. It's something you develop or end up with through blind biological bad luck.

Accordingly, there should be no more shame or stigma attached to treating depression with antidepressants than there is to a diabetic's treating her diabetes with insulin injections.

Removing stigma is a laudable goal. And to the extent that the biomedical model has succeeded in lowering the social and psychological barriers that have kept people from seeking help for mental health problems, it deserves to be praised. But portraying depression as a disease like diabetes has also served less pure, or at least more purely pragmatic, goals. I mentioned that Americans are wary of the idea of taking a medicine that only blunts the ordinary pain of living—one that allows us to bear up a little better under our problems, without really solving them. This wariness had something to do with the demise of tranquilizers, which ran afoul of the FDA, the public, and the Rolling Stones because of their image as a treatment for the stresses and strains of everyday life. By depicting them as being functionally very different from tranquilizers, the biomedical model allowed antidepressants to avoid the same fate.

The makers of SSRIs could have marketed their new products as treatments for anxiety; indeed, in the early days, some looked into it. But after the 1980s, after tranquilizer makers had been slapped on the wrist by regulators for marketing their products as remedies for everyday tension, and after stories of tranquilizer addiction had flooded the media, a different approach seemed more desirable. To ensure that SSRIs didn't end up with a "mother's little helper" reputation, their manufacturers emphasized to doctors and consumers alike that depression was a real disease with biological causes, and that SSRIs were a proper medical treatment for that disease. The psychiatrist and historian of psychopharmacology David Healy has written that by the 1990s, the same symptoms that would have once gained someone a diagnosis of anxiety neurosis and a prescription for tranquilizers was likely to be diagnosed as a mood disorder and be treated with a prescription for an SSRI.

BUT WHY EXACTLY are we so discomfited by the idea of pills that might tweak the self? Or by the thought of a drug that just slightly softens the edges of a painful world? Carl Elliott is a professor of bioethics, pediatrics, and philosophy at the University of Minnesota in Minneapolis. He writes about what he calls "enhancement technologies," interventions at the interface of medicine and self-improvement that promise "to take the edge off of some sharply uncomfortable aspects of American social life."[28] Cosmetic surgery, Prozac, Ritalin, Viagra, and Botox are all potential examples. His work provides a way of explaining the complicated feelings that antidepressants stir up for us, both as individuals and collectively.

Elliott argues that enhancement technologies fascinate and aggravate us because they alert us to a contradiction in our national value system. On the one hand, America prizes success, and life here is organized around the heated pursuit of it. America is a democracy with a high degree of social mobility; we're all searching for anything that might give us a competitive edge over our neighbors. (We are also, most likely, looking over our shoulders at whatever our neighbors might be using to get ahead, simultaneously judging them for using it, and wondering where we can get some ourselves.) On the other hand, Americans are also devoted to the idea of personal authenticity. We believe it's important to be our "real" selves and are ever fearful of losing touch with our inmost natures in the push of worldly ambition. Self-discovery and self-actualization aren't just enjoyable activities; they're social demands. In America, Elliott believes, we tend to think of life as a never-ending process of figuring out "who we are" and then striving to live in such a way that we can enact the interests and proclivities that make us unique. This focus on the self as a guiding principle may partly stem from the secular nature of our society. In America since the late nineteenth century, Elliott writes, "finding yourself has replaced finding God."[29] Being who we really are is nothing short of a moral imperative—maybe the strongest one we modern Americans have.

These two drives—on the one hand, to succeed; on the other hand, to be who you really are inside—often come into tension. Getting ahead in life is of no value if you lose yourself in the process, as any reader of *The Picture of Dorian Gray* or *A Christmas Carol* has been well advised. The possible contradiction between achieving outward success and staying true to yourself partly explains why Americans feel ambivalent about enhancement technologies, antidepressants included.

When it comes to antidepressants in particular, there's one more rumple: the American attitude about happiness. In this country, happiness is another ideal that carries nearly the weight of a moral imperative; as Elliott observes, there is an unspoken expectation in America that people should feel and act happy most of the time. Travelers to the United States often remark that in America, more than other places, cheerfulness is viewed as a default state, and that there's considerable pressure to present oneself as upbeat. There's also a peculiarly American belief that authenticity and happiness stand in a causal relationship to each other—that *really being oneself* will lead to happiness every time.

Elliott thinks that this belief evolved from a loose interpretation of Freud, who taught that unhappiness was caused by repressions of various kinds: by that logic, the least repressed, most fully realized self would be the most happy. Americans possess, says Elliott, a naive trust that achieving perfect personal authenticity, a feat summed up in the popular phrase "self-actualization," will result in the deepest possible contentment.

So: Americans are supposed to be authentic, *and* we're supposed to be happy. When happiness comes easily, this is not a problem. But for people who aren't feeling happy and are contemplating antidepressants, it can make for tough choices. Is it better to take antidepressants and be happy (but maybe inauthentic, if you believe that antidepressants can temper the self)? Or is it better to press on, authentic but not happy? Either way, you'll be failing to fulfill the script that American lore has laid out for you: be who you are, and happiness will surely and naturally follow.

There's only one way out of this bind, and it's to believe that antidepressants make you more, not less, authentic. As it happens, this is precisely the claim that Elliott finds people make about a wide variety of enhancement technologies: people use a technique to alter a certain thing about themselves, and then speak about the alteration as something that makes them into, or expresses, who they really were inside all along. (For example, recipients of sex-change operations often describe them as a way to bring the physical body in line with a deeper reality. *I always felt like a woman, and now I am one.*) In short, people who use personal enhancements often speak like Tess did when she told Peter Kramer that, off Prozac, "I am not myself."

IN FACT, THAT move is precisely the one that most direct-to-consumer advertisements for antidepressants make. Drug companies have used personal authenticity as a selling point in antidepressant advertisements ever since the first commercials for Prozac began to run in professional journals. These ads are designed to allay doctors' and patients' fears that taking antidepressants will tamper with the user's unique personhood—while still maximizing the appeal of the drugs' effects.

Typically, the imagery of a direct-to-consumer antidepressant advertisement depicts people (post-treatment people, that is) enjoying a state of high effectiveness, bouncing through their everyday routines with a joie de vivre that would be the envy of anyone, clinically depressed or not. The Paxil ad at the beginning of this chapter, in which successfully treated adults hug, grin, accept graduate degrees, and speak in public with apparent calm enjoyment, is just the tip of the iceberg. Print advertisements for antidepressants from the 1990s and 2000s depict a cavalcade of mothers dandling babies, grown sons slapping fathers on the back, happy couples dancing barefoot in the grass, everyone flashing an openmouthed smile. Were these people enjoying the fruits of cosmetic psychopharmacology? It seemed likely. Thanks to Paxil (or Prozac, or Lexapro, or Effexor) they were feeling appropriately American levels of happiness, getting ahead, excelling at work and in their relationships at home.

But the language of those same ads drove home a very different point. If the images were consonant with the idea of cosmetic psychopharmacology and/or personal enhancement, the ads' wording bludgeoned us over the head with the idea that the medications were precisely *not* doing what Kramer had said they could: they weren't altering people, that is, but rather bringing them back to normal. To this day, ad campaign after ad campaign is designed to drive home the message that to take an antidepressant is to be not changed but, more precisely, *restored*. Antidepressants, the argument goes, turn you back into the person you really were all along. In other words, they don't tamper with personal authenticity; they enhance it.

The claim that antidepressants can make you more like yourself has been around for a long time. In the year 2000, an ad campaign for Prozac targeted at psychiatrists (it ran in the *American Journal of Psychiatry*) aimed to preempt any *Brave New World* associations with the product by prominently featuring a series of riffs on the phrase "Just like normal." As in: "Barb's golfing again . . . just like normal,"[30] and "Sue's playing with her kids again . . . just like normal."[31] (As if that wasn't enough on the theme of normalcy, in smaller print below a cartoon depicting the activity in question, the text continued: "Your patients count on you to help them feel normal again. You can count on Prozac to help restore normal functioning.") In other words, take a deep breath. No one is in danger of becoming the toasted-marshmallow-head figure on the cover of *Listening to Prozac*.

The association between antidepressants and normality abounds in direct-to-consumer ads too. The late-2000s motto of GlaxoSmithKline's Paxil CR was "Get Back to Feeling Like You Again." In a recent TV ad for the antidepressant Cymbalta, a voice-over accompanying a montage of exhausted-looking people intones, "Depression can turn you into a person you don't recognize. Unlike the person you used to be. Someone your kids don't understand."[32] The message is clear: to be depressed is to be not quite oneself. Taking an antidepressant can turn you back into who you really are. Doctors have been known to say the same thing to reluctant patients. Harold Koplewicz, a well-known child and adolescent psychiatrist, told me that when teenagers in his practice tell him that they don't know whether the person they are on antidepressants is really them or not, "My answer is always, 'It's always you, but it's the you you're supposed to be.'"

The claims that antidepressants can turn you back into your old self, or make you into the person you were meant to be, saturate antidepressant advertising, but they are larger than that too; they've become part of our cultural discourse about psychiatric medication. Individuals use the language of personal authenticity to talk about their own antidepressant experiences. On a web forum dedicated to personal stories about prescription drug use, a woman in her sixties writes that a few months after starting the antidepressant Celexa, "I am well again, to the extent that I never ever imagined I could get my old self back again."[33] For individuals, too, the claim that antidepressants restore the self is powerful and useful. It provides a way out of the bind that Carl Elliott's work points to, squaring the American imperative to be happy with the American imperative to be true to our innermost selves. It is also, in a sense, an unassailable claim: when Tess says that she isn't quite herself without Prozac, or when a web forum user writes that on medication, "I feel more like myself than I have in a long time,"[34] they're speaking a personal truth, something that feels deeply and intuitively right. It is difficult to argue—who better than you to say what it is to feel like yourself? Really believing in the comforting conclusion that

5 | I'VE NEVER BEEN TO ME

I n April 2008, the *New York Times* ran a column in which the psychiatrist Richard Friedman described the case of "Julie," a thirty-one-year-old woman who "had been on one antidepressant or another nearly continuously since she was fourteen." Julie had recently told Friedman that because she'd "grown up on medication," she didn't really have a sense of who she would be without it. She wondered but would never be able to gauge how the drugs might have affected her psychological development and her most basic sense of herself. Friedman reported listening with interest. "It was not," he wrote, "an issue I had seriously considered before."[1]

And yet, he realized, it could hardly be a unique one. Adolescence is the most common time of life for a first occurrence of depression.[2] And though no company or agency keeps data on how long individuals remain on antidepressant medication, we know anecdotally that usage often goes on continuously or nearly continuously for years, even decades. In my own interviews I spoke to a number of people who reported, like Julie, that they'd taken antidepressants throughout more or less their entire adolescence. Understandably, these people often asked themselves how those ten or fifteen years of antidepressant use had affected the people they had become.

Julie's question to her doctor is difficult if not impossible to answer. Friedman admits that he can't tell his patient how growing up on antidepressants affected her, except to remind her that the course of untreated serious depression is nothing to be desired. He advised readers that Julie herself, who had endured "several suicide attempts," credited antidepressants with saving her life. But even when doctor and patient both trust that antidepressants are the right choice, the existential questions that the medications raise don't just go away. For many people, they linger or recur from time to time, a significant feature of the overall antidepressant experience.

EMILY WAS TWENTY-EIGHT years old, and in the outlines of her story, she could have been Julie's twin. She had started Prozac when she was fourteen and remained on it, with only a few short breaks, ever since. Emily was raised in the Midwest by her mother and older siblings, where she attended private schools and enjoyed what she describes as a comfortable life. After college she moved to New York City and began working as a freelance writer. She has established herself well; it's entirely possible that you've read something with her byline. Her experience exemplifies many of the questions that people who come of age on antidepressants ask themselves—about what the real self is, how medication affects development, and whether or not to stay on medication as adults—as well as the ways that they arrive at personal answers to these questions.

I met Emily on one of the first crisp fall mornings of the year, at a café about halfway in between our respective neighborhoods.

In a casual, floppy sweater, with her blond hair pulled back from her face, she looked cute and cool, as if ready to audition for the part of schoolboy crush or loyal best friend. I asked her to tell me how she got started on antidepressants, and she began by describing herself as someone who felt from an early age that there was something a little different about her. "I was always sort of depressed, even as a little kid," she said. She remembered feeling tense often, "having the same crazy anxiety feeling that I have about things now, but about childhood things." She smiled self-deprecatingly. "Things that, with hindsight, I think 'That's not normal.'" In elementary school she could worry all day about the fact that she was going to have to go home and do her chore (at the time, scooping out the cat litter); the feeling of responsibility, however inconsequential, filled her with dread.

The word *paralyzed* came up a lot in Emily's stories about herself. "I remember having paralyzing nostalgia as a kid," she said. "Like being eight, and looking at pictures from when I was five, and crying." She frequently worried herself sick over things that most people go months without giving a passing thought to. In middle school, she could lie in bed and think about the universe expanding, about Earth's tiny size and relative unimportance, until human life began to feel completely pointless. "I'm saying this now laughing," she explained, "but back then it was awful. It was completely, paralyzingly scary and also just made me feel like I never wanted to do anything. What was the point of getting up?"

Around fifth grade, Emily's worries began to center more and more on schoolwork. "I was always good at school," she said, "but I would come home and spend five hours on homework that probably should have only taken me half an hour. It's not that it was too hard or anything. It would just overwhelm me, and I would obsess about it, and get really anxious. I would overthink questions until they became, I don't know, impossible meta-quandaries."

In ninth grade, Emily had a crisis. "I had mono, and it went undiagnosed for a while," she explained. "And I think that constant exhaustion, coupled with my anxiety over schoolwork, coupled with my obsession over friends and my mom being volatile—I really just lost it. I got super depressed. I think I stayed out of school for three weeks. I would run to the bathroom crying in the middle of the day." Emily's mother took her to a talk therapist, and also to a psychiatrist, who prescribed Prozac. Emily remembers not liking the idea of taking medication at first. "I was fourteen, so I didn't have a choice of whether to take it or not," she said. "I remember throwing a fit, and my mother just making me. But I think that as soon as I saw and felt the difference, I became much more okay with it."

Still, Emily's uneasiness about medication led her to go on and off Prozac a couple of times in high school. During a year spent as an exchange student in Spain, she didn't take it and felt fine; social life kept her busy, and in a foreign environment, she said, schoolwork didn't cause so much anxiety. She became more committed to antidepressants in college. "Freshman year I was off it for a while," she remembered. "And I remember in some kind of writing 101, the most basic writing class, we had to write a paragraph about some essay we'd read. And I stayed up all night writing a hundred words. Just having to be perfect—I can't even tell you. When I think about that one incident now, I am like, 'That is insane.'" That's the point at which Emily decided that she had a serious and lasting problem with anxiety around performance-oriented tasks and deadlines, particularly ones involving writing. Since that time, Prozac has been a consistent part of her routine. The medication, she finds, frees her so she can do her work and meet her obligations. She believes it allowed her to finish college without losing her mind, and that it's what facilitated her eventual choice of career. "I don't think I'd be able to be a writer without it," she said.

Even so, Emily thinks frequently about who she would be without Prozac, and whether her life might be better—or worse—if medication had never entered into it. "I do wonder," she said. "I do think Prozac has helped me a lot. But I wonder, if I'd never gotten antidepressants, who would I be? What would I be like?" She sketched out a couple of possibilities. "For all I know, I wouldn't be alive," she said. "But maybe I would also be—I mean, what would Virginia Woolf have been like if she had taken antidepressants, you know? Maybe I would be great in some other way, but I would be unhappy."

Sometimes, she worries that antidepressants block off an experience of herself that would be more intimate and direct, more "authentic." The times she quit antidepressants in high school, she said, she was motivated by "a desire to be clear and clean, to just be absolutely myself." She wonders whether, because of Prozac, she's less "in touch with my body, and my feelings" than other people. In low moments, she can make herself feel bad by wondering whether her years of antidepressant use might have had a permanent effect: "Maybe I messed with who I really am by changing my body chemistry."

Even today, Emily says that she's often beguiled by a wish to leave Prozac behind and get, as she imagines it, back in touch with herself. On the day of our conversation she was even mulling over a plan. "I've been thinking," she said. "Once I finish some articles, at the end of the year, maybe January or February, I need to take some time off work and spend some time, you know, reading, being outdoors or, you know, just to get myself—maybe that would be a time to go off Prozac and just see how it is."

But the idea of taking a medication holiday is easier said than done for Emily. Taking antidepressants, she believes, is what allows her to pursue her chosen livelihood. Writing is how Emily supports herself. Being a writer is also her identity, one she's worked hard for and that she values. "At this point, I literally feed and clothe and house myself one hundred percent through my writing," she said. "So when I think about experimenting with going off medication, the chance of writing anxiety is more worrisome to me than the depression. Even on the best days, I don't find writing to be easy. Can I really risk making it harder?" Or would she want to? Emily *feels* like a writer. It isn't just what she does; it's what she is. "I mean, I think about not writing," she continued. "But then I'm like, what would I *do*? And not even just the money. Can I really not write anymore? It feels kind of like a dead end."

Emily thinks that she could get by without antidepressants, but that to do so she'd have to reorganize her life and probably sacrifice her profession. She told me she's read about people who have "structured their lives to avoid any kind of stress," and she said, "I have to think that would work. If I were doing something completely different, that didn't require the sorts of tasks that usually cause problems for me, I think I could be fine without medication." As an example, she thinks back to that exchange-student year in Spain. The fantasy of remaking her life into one of less-challenging work and no medication can be tempting, an incursion of the romantic critique of antidepressants into Emily's inner dialogue about herself and her choices. "So I think about that sometimes," she continued. "Maybe if I just worked in a café and made that my life. Maybe that's the answer."

And yet, and yet. There are two strains that run though our conversation, like different instrument sections in an orchestra, balancing each other out. As much as Emily wonders who she'd be without medication—and clearly these questions are very active for her—she also defends the authenticity and the validity of the person she has become. This second voice talks against the first voice, and against the voices of people in her life who call Emily's antidepressant use into question. "Sometimes I have this feeling like I failed," she said. "I have this one friend who says things to me like, 'You've just never learned to deal with your problems.' And most of the time I don't agree with that, but there are times when I think, 'God, maybe he's right. Maybe instead of really dealing with the problems, I've chosen to go the weaker route.'" She nudged a crust of French toast around her plate with her fork. "But then again, it seems to me like maybe medication *is* a way of dealing with it. It's a way of making what can be a tough choice. I could choose not to take it and have living without it be what I focus on, but in the end I stay on it because there are other things in my life, there are other problems and issues where I'd rather concentrate my energy."

At twenty-eight, Emily still asks herself regularly how fourteen years on antidepressants have affected the person she's become. There is much she doesn't know. Would she be a better, if more tortured, writer without medication? Would a simpler life without Prozac, if she could achieve it, have more meaning? Who *is* she, really: the adult she's made herself into, or the unmedicated person she's only met a few times since adolescence? Or is that distinction an illusion? There are also some things that she does feel certain about, such as that medication keeps her perfectionism to a manageable level, lets her live the life she's used to and do work that she values. Tentatively, she's answered her ambivalence about antidepressants by affirming that the identity that she's created on them, and which they support, is more real and more valuable than the hypothetical identities she imagines she might have if she were not taking antidepressants.

But her struggle has been an active one, and the existential questions that antidepressants raise for her are still there in the background, occasionally demanding reconsideration. With Emily, as for many people who have grown up on antidepressants, these questions—sharp and uncomfortable at some moments, barely perceptible at others—are now woven tightly into the fabric of her life.

THOSE EXISTENTIAL QUESTIONS are felt more keenly by some people than by others. One thing that causes variance is a person's sense of how ill they are. People who strongly and viscerally believe in their own need for medication are less likely to spend time and energy second-guessing about the self that might have been. Emily, for example, believes that she'd be able to get along without antidepressants in a life rinsed of professional stress. So from time to time, she feels compelled to weigh the value of the career she has built for herself against the strength of her desire to live without medications. For other people, the questions break down very differently. Those who believe that antidepressants literally have life-saving power often find it easier to accept antidepressants as, on balance, an element of good in their lives, and move on.

This is the equation that Claire makes. Now thirty-four, Claire went through periods of depression in high school, and then again after dropping out of college. When she was in her early twenties, a psychiatrist put her on an SSRI, and she found it helpful. Six months later, Claire's brother, who had been suffering from undiagnosed mental illness, killed himself. After his death, stories of other mental illness in the family began to come out. "That gave me a really different perspective on taking antidepressants," Claire said. "Since then, I have tried to take my mental health very seriously," a commitment that has included staying on medication, out of a sense that she is at high genetic risk. Once in a while, Claire wonders whether she really needs antidepressants. When we talked, she was in the process of finalizing a divorce. She said she was managing well, but had speculated about whether antidepressants were preventing her from digesting the experience: "Am I numbing myself by taking medication?" she asked. "Would I process things more quickly if I were feeling them on a deeper level?" But when she thinks about quitting, she always remembers her brother, her perception of her own vulnerability, and her feeling that over the years, medication has helped her a lot. She told me that while she doesn't agree with the analogy comparing depression to a physical disease in every case, she does think it applies in her own. "For me, okay, my brother killed himself," she said. "The issue is pretty cut-and-dried. It's probably safer to medicate."

The matter is even clearer for Josh. Of all the people I spoke to for this book, Josh corresponded most closely to my preconceptions about what a person with clinical depression might sound like. His voice on the phone line had a flatness to it that I desperately wanted to cheer up. Josh, who is thirty-two, told me that his father had committed suicide when Josh was four. One of his uncles also committed suicide, and his mother and both his brothers suffer from depression. Josh made a suicide attempt of his own when he was fourteen, an event that led to his first prescription for an antidepressant. He told me matter-of-factly that he remembers feeling "disappointed" that his attempt hadn't succeeded, but that after it, he became "resigned to living." Josh did start feeling better on medication, and has continued to take it since. He said that while he still doesn't consider himself to be remarkably happy, he knows that antidepressants keep him out of the depths of depression. "I'm confident that I'm not going to kill myself," he said, adding, "I'm very aware of how it feels to be a survivor of suicide. I didn't want to put my family through that again."

I asked Josh whether he ever wrestled with feeling that antidepressants might prevent him from knowing who he really is, and he says that hardly matters to him. "I can understand that," he said. "I felt that a little bit. But, yeah, it doesn't really enter into it. I've probably been off them about four times, and when I do, my life will slowly slide into just, I'm just miserable. The last time, when I was represcribed them, they said that the more times you have to go back on—they just said that I might be one of those people who needs to be on it, and I agreed." He told me he has an ex-girlfriend who once wondered "if medication was affecting my ability to feel love. And I don't know. But it's not—it's not a choice of being in love or—I mean, I need to be on it. I can't go off it to figure out if I can bond more strongly without them."

When you need the pills the way he does, says Josh, the question of personal authenticity "becomes kind of moot." Josh is pretty sure that antidepressants are what keep him alive. At this point, taking them "is just kind of part of who I am."

There is also a sizable group of people for whom antidepressants simply *don't* raise troubling questions about personhood. David Ramirez, a psychologist and the director of counseling and psychological services at Swarthmore College, says that the young adults he sees in his practice reliably break down into two groups. "For some people, it's like 'Whatever, it's like a vitamin, I just take it,'" he said. Others brood. "For other people, it's like, 'I am this person who's also on this medication, but maybe there's this other person I could be, who I don't know who that is. I don't know who I would be if I wasn't on this.' Some people feel more realized on medication, and that's nice," he said. "Other people feel unrealized." Ramirez thinks that these responses are rooted in differences of character: some people are just inclined to feel that taking an antidepressant is a philosophical dilemma, and some aren't.

Perhaps not surprisingly, a majority of the people who answered my call for interviews were the brooding type—at least to a degree. But some of those I talked to contrasted themselves with people they've known who have taken antidepressants without angst:

I was in a relationship for a while with a guy who was also on antidepressants. But he wasn't in therapy or anything, never had been. He just woke up and took a pill every day. It drove me crazy—how can you not want to know what's really going on? But he just didn't care to think about it. And that was certainly his choice. But it wasn't one I could have made.   —*Vivian, age twenty-four*

I have a friend who's been on Prozac since she was really little, and she has always said "No, there's just this chemical thing in my brain, and I take my happy pills and I'm good." And her depression really has been helped by taking medication, so she doesn't think there's anything behind it except maybe a genetic tendency to some sort of brain malfunction.

—*Elizabeth, age twenty-five*

By a similar token, Teresa, the twenty-five-year-old in Iowa, wrote of feeling so certain that her depression was "other" that she never doubted that antidepressants reveal her authentic self. "For me, I always felt like the *depression* hid who I really was," she wrote. "My therapist commented earlier today on how much I'd changed since she started working with me, and I was confused. To me, I haven't changed at all. I've just shed the tremendous weight of depression and anxiety that was stifling my actual personality."

BUT MOST OF the people I talked to did wonder, sometimes with a fair amount of torment, how antidepressants had impacted who they are, and how they experience the world and themselves in it. It makes sense that they did: developmental psychologists agree that establishing an identity is the main developmental task of adolescence (a stage that spans, roughly, the ages eleven to nineteen years), and adolescents who are already actively reflecting on questions of identity are likely to fold medication into the process. "Teenagers tend to incorporate their use of medication into their identity and reflect on its meaning more than adults," said Lara Honos-Webb, a Walnut Creek, California–based clinical psychologist. "Because teens are presented with the question of 'Who am I?,' being a person who takes medication gets included in that quest." Sharing some of their comments can illuminate what this kind of wondering sounds and feels like.

One of the ways that teens can incorporate using antidepressants into their developing identities is to internalize the idea that they're sick. Honos-Webb has noticed this phenomenon in her practice. "I think what's tragic, and I think this is what a lot of psychiatrists really miss, is that the diagnosis and the medication have a serious risk that a teenager will define themselves as fundamentally flawed and lacking," she told me. "I have seen teenagers directly say, 'Why should I try, if I'm already handicapped in some way?'" And though that isn't the message that anyone would want a young person to take away from treatment, I talked to a number of people who remember hearing it that way.

Natalie, twenty-four, started taking antidepressants at age thirteen, followed quickly by stimulant medications for ADHD. She said that she was having real trouble and that her parents wanted to help. "But when you put someone on a drug that early, it automatically puts in the kid's head, and it put in my head, that there was something *wrong* with me," she told me.

And so it just caused me to feel like I didn't belong, or that I was mentally unstable. They kept telling me that, and after a while you start to believe it, and you're all fucked-up. And you know, you can't hang out with people because you think you're too fucked-up. —*Natalie, age twenty-four*

Alexa said she believes that taking antidepressants in middle school made her self-define as a sad person to such an extent that she actually avoided developing her identity in other areas. Her comment reminded me of something else that Honos-Webb told me—that though antidepressants are effective at managing negative emotions, they don't in themselves provide the sense of meaning and direction that a person equally needs in order to find her way in life. Alexa thinks that in her own case, medication made that direction harder to find. "I think that one of my criticisms is really [of prescribing] antidepressants for kids," Alexa said.

Just because your identity isn't formed yet, and to a certain extent I feel like you have to play catch-up. Because even if you grow up and become an adult like everyone else, if you go off them, there's just this cloud of wonder about "What am I really like?" Those are the cheesy questions that you ask yourself when you're a teenager. And I didn't really ask myself those questions. I was just like "Oh, I'm someone who's sad, because I'm on these drugs." And so for me, I feel like it limited me. Like I didn't really explore myself.

—*Alexa, age twenty-three*

On the other hand, not everyone who took antidepressants felt that it had a negative impact on their identity. Dana, now thirty-one, grew up in Boulder, Colorado. Her parents divorced when she was ten, and she started going to therapy around that time. She described herself as a moderately depressed high-school student: "I always maintained functionality," she said. "My grades weren't dropping. I was always a solid student and a solid member of my family. But I was definitely showing signs of depression. I was definitely hurting, and seeking something to make me not feel the way I felt." At fifteen, she asked to be examined by a psychiatrist. She was hoping to get a prescription for medication, both to feel better, and because something about the idea of being on medication appealed to her. "One of my best friends at the time had ended up on Prozac," she said, "and I remember starting to feel a little jealous, like it sort of legitimized her experience a bit more than mine. There wasn't no reason for me to consider it—I was certainly a sad, alienated kid—but she sparked the idea." Dana saw a psychiatrist through her mother's health plan, had "the really brief diagnostic interview," and came away with her own prescription for Prozac.

Perhaps in part because she had pushed to do it, Dana said, she never felt uneasy about taking antidepressants. She also couldn't relate to friends on antidepressants who used to worry about whether the pills would change who they were. "I couldn't really empathize with that," she told me. "That hadn't been a fear of mine, and it hadn't been my experience. Probably because [taking Prozac] was my idea. Nobody said, 'You're too messed up, you need to start taking these pills.' I kind of asked to do it, and in a way I asked to do it to validate my existence and my experience, so it makes sense to me that I had the opposite reaction. Actually, I felt a little proud of it." To Dana, being on antidepressants was a way of taking herself seriously and distinguishing herself from other people—marking herself as a certain kind of person in the almost tribal milieu of high school. "I played high school volleyball," she explained,

and I was definitely not the sort of person you would associate with a volleyball team. And I remember, I have a memory of sort of intentionally taking my Prozac in front of some members of the team, and I think it was a little bit like, "Just to be clear here, I'm not quite like you guys." There was a little bit of "Yes, what this means about me is that I'm a deeper feeler, and I'm kind of a tortured soul"—you know, whatever a fifteen- or sixteen-year-old might like to own about a depressed persona, I embraced, because it kind of set me apart. Maybe I already felt apart, and it was a way to own it, like "Yeah, fuck you, I *am* different."

Taking Prozac became part of her identity, but it was a part she actively welcomed.

Even so, when Dana looks back, she does believe that antidepressants reinforced her sense of herself as a depressed person, and she sometimes wonders whether that reinforcement strengthened what depressive tendencies she did have—whether those tendencies would have weakened or worked themselves out in time. "I don't question the feelings that I had as a teenager," she said. "But I don't know if I needed meds at the time, or if someone could have said to me, 'Hey, why do you think you need Prozac?' and that could have been a different kind of conversation." She continued: "I felt that [Prozac] maybe solidified my depression a little bit, made it something more reified and substantial, rather than letting it fall away."

Some young people who take antidepressants dwell on their inability to know whether what they are feeling is "real." Adults experience this too—"Is it me or my meds?" is a common-enough question-complaint at any age—but young adults, who have less experience telling depressed thoughts apart from nondepressed ones, and comparing the way they feel on medication to the way they feel off it, often mull over the question with special intensity.

Aaron told me that in his very affluent suburban middle school in Connecticut, psychotropic drug use was so common that "it would get to where I'd be in my school cafeteria and everyone was sort of talking about what they were on. To the point where if you weren't on something, it was just weird." So he didn't feel socially judged or outcast when he started taking an antidepressant at age twelve. But he did describe a persistent sense of uncertainty around his own emotions, which he associates with medication. "I've been raised on the idea that there is a chemical imbalance in my brain," he said, "and that it's also a genetic thing, because both my mother and my grandmother have been on some kind of antidepressant at certain stages of their lives." By now, he said, he's used to the idea. "But also," he continued,

"It's only chemical" is a really uncomfortable thing, because you tend to distrust your own thoughts at a certain point. Because you're not aware of whether what you're feeling is a product of a chemical imbalance, or an actual thing. So I'm a little bit—I'm uncomfortable treating it purely as a chemical thing. —*Aaron, age twenty-two*

Aaron is familiar with the idea that his illness consists of a chemical imbalance that affects his consciousness, but he doesn't like the way the belief leads him to continually second-guess whether any given feeling he has is an "actual thing" or a product of his disease. Antidepressants, he said, just compound matters. Rather than making him trust his thoughts more, they add one more layer of complexity to the system: when he takes them, he wonders whether his feelings are "real," disordered, influenced by medication, or some combination of all three. In this culture, we're supposed to be aware of our true feelings and use them as a guide to action. Aaron doesn't believe he's able to do that in a straightforward way, and the thought pains him. "For a long time, I looked into 'anything but pills,'" he said, explaining that he was motivated by his wish to avoid the question that medications always raise for him: "How can I really know whether what I'm feeling is genuine?"

Sophia began to take antidepressants after being diagnosed with anorexia at age thirteen. The medication, along with a therapy program for teenagers with eating disorders, seemed to help, but Sophia resented having to be on medication—not least because it made her feel as though she couldn't know who she would be or what she would be feeling without it.

I went through high school with very frequent treatments. I was at doctors three times a week; it was my main extracurricular activity. Much to my resentment at the time. All through high school I was on the drugs, and I couldn't tell whether they were doing anything, but I was on a high enough dose that I was scared to go off. I didn't know what my personality would be, really, if I didn't have them, because I'd grown up with them. —*Sophia, age twenty*

Now a junior in college, Sophia still takes antidepressants. She made an attempt at quitting after her freshman year but restarted a year later when another anorexic crisis forced her to take a temporary break from school. Despite the appearance that she benefits from medication, Sophia says that she still struggles with her inability to know exactly what antidepressants are doing for her, and the impossibility of prizing apart how they fit into the bigger picture of her personality and her moods.

Now I'm still on Lexapro and kind of freaked-out about going off it, because I don't know what progress to attribute to it. Because I *am* doing better now. Drugs are very confusing.

Well, you don't have to go off it.

I know, I don't have to. But I don't even know if it's doing anything, and I don't know—there's no objective way to measure it, because if you have a good day, you feel better, and if you have a bad day, you feel worse. And I feel that's fairly normal. So how does Lexapro play into that? It's a really bizarre question, when you think about it.

And you don't like having to wonder that.

Yeah, not at all. I would prefer to know that my mental states just modulate themselves, and by themselves. I'll never know if I don't go off the meds. But when I do, if something bad happens—is that because I went off?

Sophia told me that she thinks her attitude toward antidepressants has something to do with the kind of person she is. "Some people I've talked to really trust their medications, and believe they work for them wonderfully, and are perfectly happy staying on them forever," she said. "I am rarely satisfied with my current state, so maybe I'm the kind of person who's just always going to be worried that something's not quite as good as it could be, or 'What if this isn't real,' or philosophical crises like that."

Part of Sophia's dissatisfaction with antidepressants has to do with her sense that in order to use them, she has to cede some control over her emotions, both to a drug and to the people who prescribe it. "It's confusing, especially when you're on and off medications all the time," she said, "and you're trying different ones, and people are telling you what to do, and you [ask yourself], 'Should I trust this psychiatrist who doesn't know who I am anyway?'" She's not the only person who mentioned that antidepressants make them feel as though they weren't fully in control of their own thoughts and actions, or confuse them about the degree of control they do have. Alexa told me that once she started to think of herself as depressed, every bad thing that happened began to seem like further confirmation that pills were the only thing standing between her and disaster.

> Especially when my best friend tried to kill herself. I was like, "Is that going to happen to me?" I just started losing a sense of my own willpower. In a way, my biggest problem with being on drugs was like this lack of self-esteem, because you don't really know that you're in control of your life.
>
> —*Alexa, age twenty-three*

Still others associate antidepressants with a sense of unknowing that can last even after the medication itself is withdrawn. Jessica, twenty-four, who started antidepressants in fifth grade and took them up through her second year in college, feels less conflicted about her antidepressant use than a number of the other people I talked to. "I'm cool with who I am now, having been on all those things," she told me. But she voiced a feeling that many of those who started antidepressants at a young age echoed, a simple but touching sense of not being certain how medication contributed to the person she became. During her high school years, Jessica remembered,

> people, various friends or boyfriends at the time asked me—because I've always been very open about [taking medication]—people have asked me, "Do you think it interferes with your personality, or your ability to know yourself? Is it somehow stopping what would naturally come forward?" And I felt okay at the time. So I kind of said, "No," but I wasn't quite sure. And honestly I'm still not sure.

IT WOULDN'T BE right to end our tour of the topic of antidepressants and the teenage self without mentioning one final, very concrete way in which antidepressants can affect a developing identity, and that's in the realm of sexuality. SSRIs are well known for causing "sexual side effects," a catchall term for a broad range of occurrences in both men and women—ranging from loss of interest in sex, to difficulty performing, to delay in orgasm or inability to have an orgasm at all. Sexual side effects were originally touted as rare with the SSRIs, but some studies have shown that they affect over half the people who take the medications.[3]

For adults, sexual side effects are undeniably a nuisance; sometimes they can be among the biggest drawbacks of the drugs. For teens, they're also a nuisance, with one added dimension. Just as teens don't have a sense of their baseline adult personality with which to judge whether and how antidepressants may be affecting them, teens also lack a baseline impression of their own sexuality. Adults who are familiar with their own sexual norms will have an easy time knowing when those norms have been upset. But for adolescents who are just growing into their sexuality, the picture can be more mysterious.

Sexual side effects from SSRIs haven't been widely discussed in the context of teenagers, possibly out of a cultural ambivalence about whether adolescents should be sexually active or not. But because SSRIs influence not just performance but also a person's thoughts and desires, these side effects are relevant for teens who aren't having sex as well as for those who are. In the article in which he described his patient Julie, Richard Friedman mentioned a woman in her mid-twenties who came to him complaining that she often felt pressured by her boyfriend for sex. "I've always had a low sex drive," she explained. Friedman pointed out that the young woman had been taking an SSRI since her mid-teens; she had "understandably mistaken the side effect of the drug for her 'normal' sexual desire and was shocked when I explained it," he wrote. Timothy Dugan, a child and adolescent psychiatrist at Harvard's Cambridge Hospital, told me he thinks that the question of SSRIs' effects on young adult sexuality deserves consideration, especially in light of the importance that sexuality plays in psychological theories of development. "If Freud's right, then sexuality should drive development, and drive connections with other people," he said. "If you've taken the edge off [with a medication], then what's that about? There are real side effects that have, in my mind, real or potential developmental impact."

When I started to ask people about their experiences, I found many who said or suspected that medication had influenced their sexuality, though a number of them didn't make this connection until later—and some still aren't completely certain. Laura, a twenty-three-year-old graphic designer who took Zoloft as a teenager, said: "I was an arty senior in a big suburban high school." When it came to sex, "I just wasn't interested. I thought it was the Zoloft. But, again, I wasn't sure." Alexa said she didn't really blossom sexually until after she quit medication at twenty. "On those drugs," she said, "I had no sexual—I didn't even know if I was straight!" Aaron also says he experienced sexual side effects from medication. "Now that I think about it," he wrote in an e-mail, "there may be a correlation between [the times during college] when I was on medication, and when I wasn't getting laid. I wouldn't have much of a sex drive on medication, and there were times when I just didn't have the ability to perform." And Emily told me in our conversation that "the sex thing" is definitely part of her occasional desire to go off antidepressants. When I asked her to explain, she said, "I think that I have a really healthy sex drive, but it's impossible for me to know. Even if I do go off it, my brain has formed around these chemicals now for that last half of my life. I mean, I started having sex when I was taking antidepressants! So I'm never going to be clear on what the difference would have been."

Others had a clearer sense of what was happening. Dana, who started taking Prozac at fifteen, was aware of some sexual side effects at sixteen, and then lost her ability to have an orgasm the following year. The situation was "frustrating, and depressing in its own right," but she understood the reasons for it. She shared her concerns with her psychiatrist, who switched her to Wellbutrin, a non-SSRI antidepressant with a lower incidence of sexual side effects. Dana dealt with the problem well—and increased awareness may help more teenagers and young adults to do the same—but others may remain too embarrassed to ask for help, or will lack a basis to notice the difference the drugs are making.

NOT ALL, BUT a considerable number of adolescents who take psychiatric medications find that these medications impact their search for an identity. They feel that the drugs make the question "Who am I?" more complicated to answer. They may struggle with the feeling that the answer to the question could be something negative: "I'm someone who's sick, because I take these drugs." Or they worry that the medication alienates them from their real emotions: "How can I really know if what I'm feeling is genuine?" Over time, they may come to feel that the selves they know are not, somehow, their real selves, or not the selves they might have been: "I didn't know what my personality would be without it, really, because I'd grown up on it." Even people who end up affirming their choice to take medication live with these questions, and can feel a need to reconsider them from time to time: "I do wonder. If I'd never gotten antidepressants, who would I be? What would I be like?"

It's easy to laugh at the concept of being "genuine," or roll your eyes at the idea of the real self. In fact, sometimes it's hard to take these notions with a straight face. Alexa remembered asking herself, "What am I really like?" but she also knowingly referred to it as "one of the cheesy questions you ask yourself when you're a teenager." In the academy, scholars have been declaring for decades that the true self is dead. For the last twenty years, the dominant academic theories of personhood have focused not on the idea of essence but on performance and changefulness, the sense that we don and doff identities at will as we move through our lives. Intellectually, we all know that the true self is more of a metaphor than a literal reality—we don't really believe that there is some perfectly realized version of each of us hovering out there, just waiting to be discovered like a vein of gold.

But no matter how well we understand the academic critique of the essential self, or how much we feel disposed to dismiss "Who am I?" and its ilk as "cheesy questions," most of us still want to feel, in some way, like ourselves. We may never achieve the highly concrete answer to the question of who we are that we first imagine possible as young teenagers—but a notional sense of self is something that we all rely on from day to day. This sense doesn't have to be as well-defined as words like *genuine* and *authentic* can make it sound, but we need to be able to trust it intuitively. Such a workaday sense of who we are is a necessary value, one that guides us in our choices and informs our relationships with other people and with our world.

Knowing that many adolescents at least perceive antidepressants as making a reliable sense of self harder to find is important. A feeling of authenticity is, admittedly, an intangible thing to lose—but in a society that still prizes a notion of authentic selfhood, however problematic, it can also be a significant one. The fact that antidepressants can frustrate the adolescent search for identity isn't a comprehensive argument against their use in youth, of course. Every expert I talked to, from the most bullish on medication to the most conservative, agreed that depression in adolescence can be devastating and that antidepressants are sometimes the best response. (Untreated mental disorder can itself have a negative impact on a young person's developing identity.) But the sense of uncertainty and self-estrangement that Aaron, Sophie, Emily, Julie, and many others in their situation attribute to medication is powerful. Even when they decided that the benefits of being on antidepressants outweighed the detriments, they often felt that they had lost a direct way of relating to themselves that they imagined other people their age to possess. That sense of loss, they said, is stubborn and real. For many, it is a central and long-lasting feature of the experience of growing up on antidepressants, and it is one that deserves to be taken into account when we are weighing the decision of whether to put young people on psychoactive drugs that they may use and develop with for years.

6 | TWO RED CHAIRS

Just about everything I own in the world is bouncing down route 81 in the back of my father's silver Toyota pickup truck. I'm trailing him in my own Honda Civic, and from time to time I can catch part of my material life—an armchair with red cushions, the mattress we bought this morning at an Ikea in New Jersey—flash into view when the blue tarp tied across the truck bed flaps in the wind. Road conditions are what my high school driver's ed teacher would have deemed poor. The gray clouds that moved in as we passed through Scranton have begun to shed fat drops of rain that burst on contact like grade-school spitballs. My father is speeding, and I'm driving faster than feels safe to keep up with him, cursing under my breath. The speeding and cursing help distract me from the uncomfortable thought that sinks in a little further with each passing mile: *I'm really doing this. This is really real.*

We are headed to Ithaca, New York, where I'm supposed to start my first year as a PhD student in English at Cornell University. But it feels as if I'm driving off the edge of one of those medieval maps of the world, into a void where sea monsters wait to swallow lost sailors.

THAT MORNING IN Brooklyn, I hugged good-bye to my friend Anna on the strip of grass separating the sidewalk from the street in front of our building. We had graduated from college and moved to the city together nine months before. Anna planned to stay indefinitely, while I'd already applied to schools and expected to be moving on at the end of summer, though I didn't yet know where. We rented a tiny loft near the river and built denlike bedrooms out of drywall and metal two-by-fours; in honor of my temporary-resident status, I slept on an air mattress for months. During the day I worked at a coffee shop while Anna went to her internship at a record label. In our off times, we explored our wonderful and bewildering new city, or compared notes about it while sitting together in the dusty glory of our first grown-up apartment.

As thrilling as New York could be, the new shape of social life alternately excited and dazed me. In the city we went out a lot, but people seemed to disappear back into their lives more mysteriously; there was no nucleus, no point of reference to understand ourselves in relation to. I missed the way that Portland had felt like a real community. It had been a home to me, while New York City felt like a raucous way station, a wild party in an elevator.

In the first months after college I had ended up applying to graduate schools almost by accident, out of a sense that the real world was too baffling and amorphous to handle. I hadn't figured out what to do with my life, but I had been good at my major, English, and when one of my professors suggested that I might apply for PhD programs, the thought appealed to me. The implicit praise appealed to me too. All my life I had been a good student, adept at pleasing teachers and used to warming myself by the glow of the approval they gave me. Losing that old system for feeling worthwhile had been the hardest thing about leaving college. Getting back into the academic world, with its reassuring markers of achievement, seemed like a way both to feel good about myself again, and to silence the questions about what to do with my future that had become a monotonous, tormenting chorus inside my head.

So I applied. I did it even though something about the whole process felt rushed and wrong, like a bigger commitment than I was ready for. I drove my unease away with the lockstep of details: I filled out forms, gathered writing samples, and sent packets off to a dozen distant addresses. I was admitted to a couple of programs, and even though my campus visits made me feel crazy with ambivalence, I accepted one, because I didn't know what else to do and I wanted to make other people proud. And now, in my waning days in New York, every time I thought about it too hard I felt queasy. So I tried my best not to think about it at all.

One night in June, Anna and I went to a party, and once again I noticed that feeling that going out in New York so often gave me, of not gaining *traction*. I was tired of explaining to people I'd just met that I would soon be leaving, tired of trying to sound excited about a step that in truth I felt no excitement about. When we left around midnight, it was pouring rain so we decided to share a taxi home. I had been feeling on edge all night, and as the cab crept slowly through the darkened streets, with thick sheets of water enclosing its windows, the sensation deepened to an unbearable claustrophobia. At a stop sign a few blocks from home I threw some money into Anna's lap and let myself out into the night. I sprinted home and pounded up the six flights of stairs to the large, flat roof of the building, leaving foot-shaped pools of wetness behind me. Up there, the rain pasted my clothes to my body and then streamed freely through them. I was finally alone, as I had not been alone in New York City in months, and I threw fistfuls of gravel and banged my arms on the metal ladder that led up to the empty water tank, suddenly venting a fury I didn't know I had been carrying inside. I stayed up there, throwing and shouting and banging, until I was exhausted, and then I knelt on the layer of pointy stones that covered the rooftop and let rivulets of cool water trace small rivers down my skin.

The next morning I awoke on my air mattress. Pale, innocuous sunshine streamed in the window. I felt more truly calm than I had in months. The feeling stayed with me all day, and it was evening before I realized that I had missed my pill the night before. I was still taking Serzone, the antidepressant I had used for most of college. I had been taking it for so long now that I'd lost a sense of what it was doing for me; I only knew that if I missed a dose I would wake up in the middle of the night, overheated and itchy all over.

That evening I skipped it again. By the time I moved away from Brooklyn, two months later, the bottle had grown dusty on the shelf. It was a risky way to quit, but after all, I reasoned, Serzone hadn't protected me from everything. I felt stuck and out of touch, and I quietly hoped that taking a break from medication might help me regain control of my life. Maybe without it I'd be able to reach back and refind that thing, that sense of purpose I knew I'd had once, but that seemed to have become lost, somewhere, during college and after.

————

WHEN WE GOT to Ithaca, my father helped me carry my things up to the apartment I'd rented, sight unseen, a cozy studio on the third floor of a huge Victorian house near the edge of town. The skies were lake-effect gray, but the rain had stopped. He headed off to a motel for the night, and I sat there amid my unassembled Ikea furniture, feeling a sense of despair and a sense of unreality. We had breakfast the next morning at a greasy-spoon café, and then he drove off and left me to settling in.

On my own I found the gym and the grocery store, went to a departmental party, and tracked down the academic adviser I'd been assigned to, a woman whose facial features I no longer remember, whose office was at the end of a serpentine hallway in the Grecian building that housed the English Department. She helped me with forms. Taking care of business was rewarding in a way, but the feelings of disconnection and guilt that had broken free near the end of my time in New York were stubborn; they sat on my shoulders like birds and cawed into my ears. "This isn't actually my life," I wrote on a long document I'd started on my computer to keep track of my thoughts, in plain contradiction of fact.

A few days after arriving in town, I met my downstairs neighbor, Casey, who was a librarian at Cornell's labor school and liked to play Scrabble. Through him I met *his* friends. I wrote in letters to my mom that I'd gotten to know a librarian, a chicken farmer, a coffee shop employee, and a filmmaker. Making friends helped immensely, but my thoughts and feelings were still all tangled up. I missed New York. Ithaca seemed so small and remote and countrified. Being at school—in a funded program, no less—was an honor, but I couldn't seem to get excited about it, and that lack of enthusiasm made me feel appalled with myself. One by one

I had made all the choices that got me here, but when I opened my eyes each morning, I felt the panic of someone waking up in an unfamiliar room. The feelings didn't fade, and after a few weeks I felt worn out by the effort of trying to hide them. One afternoon I walked into the campus medical building and asked directions to the wing for mental health.

The psychiatrist I was assigned to had a difficult-to-pronounce last name, so everyone simply called her "Dr. Barbara." Dr. Barbara styled her gray hair in a bob and wore sensible, loose long dresses made of jersey knits. She hung Balinese masks on the wall of her office, and her shelves were lined with interesting books. After I began to feel better, I used to try during our appointments to imagine her at home; for some reason, I usually pictured her standing on tiptoe, filling a bird feeder. Dr. Barbara worked methodically, even more so than other prescribers I'd known. At every appointment she took me through the same few sets of questions, noting my responses in a binder. In one of her assessments she would read out statements to which I was to reply: "All of the time," "Most of the time," "Some of the time," or "Never or almost never." I still remember that one of these statements was: "I feel punished." I remember it because it was such a perfect evocation of exactly the way I did feel. She asked me practical questions too, about caffeine, alcohol, and sleep. Our appointments were brief, but she had a certain personal warmth, and I liked her and felt that she wished me well.

Dr. Barbara told me that Serzone had been pulled off the market after having been shown to cause liver damage in a few rare cases. She did think that I was depressed, though, and she recommended that I try Prozac. Prozac! Even in my low state, I was a bit excited about getting to try the oldest and most charismatic member of the SSRI family. I had told Dr. Barbara that I was having trouble feeling like getting out of bed in the morning, a symptom she seemed well familiar with and aptly called "dread of the day"; she told me that she wanted me to try Prozac in part because it has a reputation for being activating. I filled her prescription at Wegman's supermarket, took it home, and tried to think hopeful thoughts.

"ACTIVATING." BOY, WAS it ever. After a few days I felt positively wired. I couldn't sleep. I had to force myself to eat. (Dr. Barbara dutifully wrote "anorexia" in her notes, in her clear hand.) She took me down to a smaller dose and then brought me up again slowly, hoping I'd acclimate.

But I never did. During the Prozac period, I drove to Massachusetts for a party to celebrate my Uncle David's sixtieth birthday. My parents and David's children and a couple of my other aunts and uncles were meeting up at David's small farmhouse in the Berkshires. I liked it out there and was happy to go; I thought that a couple days away from Ithaca might be good for me. What I remember, though, is this: I'm in an upstairs bedroom at David's, where I've been assigned to spend the night. There is a tall four-poster bed fitted with scratchy wool blankets. It's nighttime, and I think that I might be losing my mind. I feel as if I want to molt my skin, or climb up the walls like a praying mantis and peel the wallpaper into strips with my teeth. I have never been so anxious or so uncomfortable in my entire life; I'm sweating and shaking like a Hollywood representation of someone coming off of hard drugs. I want to wake somebody else up and tell them how insanely wrong I feel, and I'm held back only by the knowledge that they won't be able to help me, and the fear that the words that would come out of my mouth might not make any sense at all.

Back in Ithaca, I called Dr. Barbara as soon as I could. She told me that it was the Prozac that had made me feel that way; that in fact it was Prozac that had had me feeling anxious and creepy-crawly for the past few weeks. The formal name for the state is akathisia, she said, and it can occur in some people who take SSRIs. This explained some of my diary entries. Looking back over recent ones, I read: "Prozac seems to make me jumpy, confused, more anxious rather than less"; a few days later I'd noted, "I feel like I am losing my shit." At David's house I'd written that on the drive out I felt "so fucked-up . . . so discombobulated it's almost frightening." Things were "too intense, cycling fast between okay and unbearable." On October 19, 2003: "I feel worlds better since the end of the Prozac adventure," and am happy to be out of "Prozac hell."

The next year, a series of emotionally-charged hearings in Congress about whether or not SSRIs can cause suicidal thoughts and behaviors in children would hinge on those drugs' ability to cause an agitated state. After analyzing the data available from clinical trials, the FDA concluded that youth on SSRIs appeared to be about twice as likely to become suicidal as those treated with placebos.[1] SSRI suicidality (which includes both "suicidal ideation" and actual attempts) occurred in about 4 percent of children and adolescents treated with the drugs,[2] while other adverse reactions, including agitation and erratic behavior, were about six times that common.[3] In 2004, the FDA required drug makers to place a "black box" warning label on SSRI antidepressants, indicating that the medications may increase the risk of suicidal thoughts and actions in children and adolescents. In

2006, it expanded the warning to include young adults up to age twenty-five.

Despite the FDA's mandate, the answer to the question of whether the SSRIs can cause suicide is still not entirely clear; the amount of data is finite, and what exists is difficult to interpret.[4] At the very least, any claims about the drugs' harmful effects have to be balanced against the fact that antidepressants do a great deal of good for many people who are or are at risk of becoming suicidal. Still, I felt rattled by my Prozac experience. No antidepressant had ever made me feel jumpy before, and I was surprised that they could, and how marked those feelings could be. I hadn't become suicidal, but the sensations the drug had given me were scary. It wasn't hard for me to imagine that if the discomfort had been worse or gone on for longer, or if my depression had had a more self-destructive cast to begin with, those feelings could have helped nudge me to do something I didn't mean to do.

Dr. Barbara took me off of Prozac immediately, and I felt better within a couple of days. Only when withdrawing from it did I get a glimpse of Prozac "working" as it left my system. For a day or two I felt like a bird that's caught a pocket of good air and is able to glide a little. The fear machine quieted down, and I was able to feel myself in the here and now: the hot coffee in the cup, the edge of the Scrabble tiles, the powdery pages of a library book.

Around Halloween, Dr. Barbara got me started on a different SSRI called Lexapro. Aware of the problem we'd had with Prozac, she instructed me to take tiny amounts: a quarter of a pill, or an eighth. Still, I couldn't eat in the mornings. My jeans began to float away from my waist, an outcome I wasn't totally unsatisfied with, although the whole experience was beginning to make me feel a bit like a science experiment. I developed headaches that Dr. Barbara sent me to a different doctor to treat. I began to resent her a little. In late November, she declared that I "wouldn't tolerate" Lexapro and wanted to try me on Paxil, but I couldn't take it anymore. I told her I wanted plain old Zoloft again, and she wrote me a prescription.

But I decided to wait some time before having it filled. As the weeks went by, life did become more manageable. I went home for winter break, wrote the papers I needed to write, returned to school, and threw a party with my neighbor Casey, an upstairs-downstairs party in both of our apartments. I made an appetizer out of roasted red peppers and smoked trout, and we served sparkling wine. My tiny apartment bustled with warm bodies, eating and laughing. After everyone went home I had a final drink with Casey at my kitchen table, and we hashed over the night: who'd come, what they'd said, who'd flirted with whom. I felt a wave of gratitude wash over me: *I came here with nothing a semester ago. And look at all this now. I have friends, I have a life.*

EVENTUALLY I DID start taking the Zoloft. It worked as it had before, making me feel calmer, brighter, and stronger. But perhaps in a fit of pique at the profession of psychiatry for the things it had put me through without so much as an "Oops, I'm sorry," I also did something that was new for me. I decided to call a real, "talk" therapist. Cornell's mental health coverage was generous and allowed for students to work with private therapists off campus. Dr. Barbara furnished me with a list of people who were accepting new patients, and I decided to pick one on the basis of whose voice I liked best on their answering-machine message. Very late at night, when I was sure no one would pick up the phone, I called every doctor's office and listened. One sounded abrasive, another sleepy, but there was a third I took a liking to right away. He spoke at the easy pace of someone who is used to choosing his words carefully, and his voice had an ever-so-slightly nasal quality that I immediately found comforting. His name was John, and in the middle of the night, I left my name and number on his machine.

The next day I was eating a lunch of soup at home, watching tiny snowflakes fall out of the gray sky and drift across the traffic light beneath my window that, being close to the edge of town, turned from green to red and back again many times without spying a car, when the phone rang.

"Hello," said a comforting, slightly nasal voice at the other end. "This is John." He told me there had been a cancellation that afternoon, and that he could see me in an hour, if I wanted to. I squeaked. John said he would understand if I wasn't ready to come so soon, since it could take some mental preparation. "But," he added, "if you're up to the challenge—"

I'd been preparing to backpedal, but at this mention of challenges my competitive streak lurched awake. "Well," I found myself saying, "if it's a *challenge*—okay, why not? I'll see you in an hour." Thirty minutes later I was bundled up and walking down Cayuga Street toward the center of town.

John's office was on the second floor of a brown brick building that had once been a school. Its lowest story holds businesses with the hippie leanings that Ithaca is known for: a health food co-op, a serious bookstore, a shop where you can buy a hammer dulcimer and a rainbow wind sock. At exactly 2:00 P.M.

John opened the door of his little waiting area and invited me into a spacious room with high ceilings, tall windows, a rug, and two dark red armchairs flanked by matching side tables with matching boxes of tissues. We sat down. He was a tall, pleasant-looking man in his forties, with comfortably shaggy brown hair and wide-set, deep blue eyes. His fashion sense ran to blues and browns, button-down shirts and sensible shoes. I liked him as much in person as I had on the phone.

John leaned forward in his chair and looked at me. He brought his hands together and then moved them apart. "So," he said. "What brings you here?"

In my journal afterward, I wrote that I'd felt like Ally Sheedy's character in *The Breakfast Club*, in the scene where she opens her enormous handbag and dumps all its contents, which are supposed to provide some glimpse inside her weird life, onto the floor. I was surprised how much can come tumbling out in fifty minutes: my angst about school, but also, unbidden, a story of how I'd made an awkward pass at the chicken farmer and how humiliated I'd felt. There were stories of the things you'd expect, like friends and family and New York, and other details that seemed to come from nowhere. John listened and made a few comments. I told him that I was studying English, and near the end of the hour he said that there was something in common between my chosen discipline and the kind of work that he did with his patients, something about the shared pursuit of narrative. He suggested that whatever made me interested in studying literature might endear me to this process as well. We agreed that I would come again, and after a few sessions, we decided to make maximum use of my insurance for the year by meeting twice a week.

sport with only one rule: you will sit in your chairs and interact.

I wasn't even quite sure what I wanted from John. Partly I wanted help with the questions that had tortured me so much when I first showed up in town: What was I supposed to be doing with my life? Had coming to grad school been the mistake that it sometimes felt like? Somehow, the idea of being a person who got depressed and took antidepressants made those questions seem harder to answer. When I felt bad, did that mean that I was doing something wrong, or was it just a symptom, best squelched or ignored? Were antidepressants helping me achieve something that was healthy and good for me, or were they preventing me from finding my way to the life I was supposed to live—a life that would suit a version of myself that didn't have to take drugs? These questions drove me wild, and I think I hoped that John could help me solve them, absolutely and forever. Most of the time, when I walked into his office with my cup of coffee, it was in the expectation of attacking one of these forbiddingly abstract topics head on. As I sank into the cushions of his red chair, though, I'd usually find myself diverted to more mundane concerns: boys I liked, my professors, my students, my family. Often I felt resentful about this, as if it were something that John, with his overwhelming interest in relationships, were *doing* to me. He was letting us get distracted from my Big Questions!

"You're really concerned with being productive, aren't you?" he said to me, sometime during our first month, when I chided us for losing sight of the target. I looked at him as though he'd just suggested that we both stand and throw money out of the window. But he had just delivered one of the first lessons of therapy, a lesson I kept getting dragged back to again and again during our two years of appointments. Our lives are made up of moments, brief interactions strung together into a whole. In a sense, the quality of a life is the aggregate quality of those moments; it is hard to be right in the entire picture of your life if you aren't right in the details. Big questions can feel unanswerable because they often are. My fantasy of an equally big solution, he was saying, was never going to work. He wanted me to start by letting go of my dream of a top-down approach, and taking a clear look at the things that were right in front of me.

Week by week, we worked our way toward a routine. I brought John little stories about my past and my present, and he responded to them. There is a stereotype out there, in movies and TV, of the maddeningly quiet therapist, who says nothing or turns every statement into a cryptic question. John wasn't quiet, though, and he wasn't cryptic. He never gave direct advice, as much as I longed for him to. But I would tell my tales and give my own commentary on situations, and sometimes John would nod and say, "That sounds right," as if he were a musician listening to a student piece and finding it harmonious.

The differences between the therapy I did in John's office and psychiatry as I'd known it were numerous and often funny. Pharmacology sessions with Dr. Barbara had always seemed amusing to me because, although they were all *about* emotion, there was no emotion in them. Especially when I was feeling all right. After she quizzed me, via multiple-choice questionnaire, about my sleeping habits, and my intake of various lawful and unlawful substances, Dr. Barbara would get to the feely part of her interview. "Any thoughts of harming yourself, or maybe not wanting to live anymore?" she would read from her paper, in a gingerly nonchalant tone of voice. The question seemed to vaguely embarrass her, and it distinctly embarrassed me. "No," I'd say heartily, feeling nothing but a wish to distance myself from this baffling hypothetical counterpart of mine who might find ordinary life so burdensome as to want a permanent way out. We'd make small talk for a minute, and then she'd hand me the prescription for the medicine that would supposedly rearrange all my innermost feelings, and I would thank her blithely and say I'd see her next time.

Psychotherapy sessions weren't just about emotion; they were full of emotion, sometimes so full as to border on the absurd. We'd sit there in our chairs like amateur astronomers on a blanket, ready to catch shooting-star emotions as they streaked across the sky. They weren't hard to catch, because they usually announced themselves with a shower of tears. What is it about therapy and crying? I cried almost every time I went in. Sometimes I cried for what seemed like the majority of the session. I laughed too, but it's the tears I remember most, leaching out of my face and into the endlessly crumbled tissues that I held in my hands. I cried when things felt good, and when they felt bad. I cried every time we began to talk about something that I wanted. I cried so much and so often that at one point I got grumpy and made a point of telling John that I wished he could hang out with me just once on the outside. *Oh yes?* he said. *What would that be like?* I told him there was more to me than tears and misgivings. "In the real world," I said, "well, you know. I'm *fun*."

WINTER GAVE WAY to a muddy, slow-starting upstate spring. Graduate coursework hadn't turned out to be as hard as I'd feared it would be. I had made friends with a group of people that included graduate students from various departments and a handful of people who weren't involved with Cornell at all. We went to the same concerts, drank at the same bar, danced after hours in one another's living rooms, and flirted and made out with each other in ever-changing though inescapably finite permutations. It was an unhurried life, and it left plenty of time to think about the work that John and I were doing. One thing that the cultural representations of therapy hadn't led me to expect was how much mental energy it takes up. Especially in the first months, therapy was always there, like a program that runs silently in the background, hogging RAM. I began to watch myself in the world with a new kind of attention, and bring to John any detail that seemed like it might help.

One of the things that lodged therapy so firmly in my mind was its new vocabulary. Psychotherapy's use of a special language is one of its most immediately obvious characteristics. It's something we use to mock therapy (when we call it "psychobabble"), and sometimes this mockery is well deserved. But deliberate language is also one of the things that makes therapy work. John specialized in regular words employed in unfamiliar ways: *collude, ward off, integrate, bear. Attachment, projection, boundaries, wish.* Learning those words and the ways in which he meant them was like learning about a whole new system of forces at work on the universe. It reminded me of being in high school physics class, catching myself thinking about gravity, acceleration, and surface friction while I did something as ordinary as brushing my teeth.

John spoke frequently of "needs" and "unmet needs," and I struggled with the meaning of these simple English terms. He asked me to consider what mine were, and I found it surprisingly hard to do. I was used to thinking about what I wanted to *achieve* down the road, or *how I wanted my life to be*, but this was different in some way that kept slipping from grasp: not about what would be impressive to me or other people, but what I really wanted, what felt good. One of the things I was curious about when I first came to therapy was relationships; I wanted to know why, after four years of serial monogamy in college, I suddenly didn't feel like I had any idea about how to relate to guys. John helped me apply the question of needs to my various entanglements, to think out whether I was getting what I wanted from the men in my life. At the time, the answer was usually somewhere between "no" and "no way," but just learning to ask the question had a revelatory value on its own.

John had a way of paraphrasing my stories back to me, so that I could really hear what I had said. Sometimes he would read between the lines, telling me about my own desires and interests as he understood them. Toward the end of our first session, he told me that I had a longing for deep personal intimacy but had had a hard time finding it. I felt like a rube at a storefront fortune-teller's shop: *Gosh, I guess I do! But how did you know?* Later, when I remarked that sometimes I longed to be back in Portland or New York, he said, "So many of the things you miss are things with people." This was so true, yet I had never put it to myself in just that way before—in the moments after he said the words, I could practically feel them being laser-engraved on my brain. I must have known on some level that connectedness made me happy, even though I had taught myself to consider time spent with other people to be time stolen from more worthy-seeming pursuits like writing or studying. But John named it, and over time that helped me to take it seriously.

I remember coming to feel as if I finally understood what therapy was. It happened when I realized that my relationship with John wasn't just an irrelevant side effect of the fact that we spent a couple hours talking every week. In the early days, I used to get impatient: John would want to remind me that I could act toward him in any way that I pleased, or would want to know how it had felt for me to run into him by accident on the streets of town, and I'd get irritated—I didn't come here, I'd think, to create yet another relationship in need of being analyzed! What I didn't understand until later was that therapy works on the premise that our lives, and our relationships, are filled with patterns, and that themes that assert themselves in the patient's other relationships will come out in the relationship with the therapist as well. The opportunity of therapy is to notice these patterns and work on them in real time, using the unusually structured affiliation between the therapist and the patient as a tool.

One day I went into his office and said to John, "Working on self-hate feels like trying to scratch my left elbow with my left hand."

"Katherine," he said, "that's why there are two of us."

IN THE END, therapy isn't as formless as the pop culture version of it sometimes makes it seem to be. It's not just a sea of "say how you feel." You do say how you feel, but over time all that talking and feeling, all that Kleenex, add up to a surprisingly logical activity. You are looking for patterns and trying to puzzle them out. Why is the experience of desire, for you, always followed by shame? Why does disappointment lead to self-hate, as reliably as a rifle shot generates a kickback? Therapy is about noticing these chains of emotion and working back through them link by link to figure out what's going on.

As I went through this process with John, a wonderful change started to take place. For the first time ever, I began to seriously consider the possibility that I might make sense. As we put the basic pieces of the system in place, I realized that there were some things that were true whether I was on medication or not. Connection made me happy. Transitions were hard. I realized how many of my depressions had come at times when structure—school, a relationship, a job—was withdrawn, severing many familiar routines in one swoop. I started to appreciate that if I did certain things (spend time with a good friend, go to the gym, say "no" to obligations I didn't really have time for), I'd feel better, and if I did other things (spend too much time without seeing people, pile on more commitments than I could manage in a certain span of time, indulge my crush on that emotionally vacant guy), I'd feel worse. Feelings, even my feelings, were subject to their own rules of cause and effect.

DURING MY SECOND year in Ithaca, blundering around in the dimly lit stacks of Cornell's graduate library, I stumbled across a book that would give me a more refined way of thinking about the magic that was happening in John's office. Karen Horney was a German psychoanalyst who emigrated to the United States in the 1930s. I hadn't heard of her, and I'd been looking for something else when I found her book *Neurosis and Human Growth* wedged into a bottom shelf next to some of the heavyweights of twentieth-century psychology, but its strange old title called out to me, and on a whim I took it home.

Horney's premise was that, in childhood, most people suffer from the feeling of being small and powerless in a dangerous world; she considered the feeling so common that she called it "basic anxiety." She believed that children attempt to soothe their fears and insecurities by resorting to their imaginations, beginning to picture a version of themselves that embodies all the traits that the child, or the people around her, find most admirable. By adolescence, these imaginings begin to solidify into the image that Horney calls the "ideal self." Our ideal selves are the smartest, the kindest, the shrewdest, the most lovable— depending on how we want to see ourselves. But what starts out as a protective fantasy quickly becomes an instrument of self-torture too, giving rise to the tricky system of inner conflicts and secondary insecurities that Horney called neurosis. Specifically, she wrote, neurotics suffer from the strain of their own doomed quest to become the superhuman image they have created. They flagellate themselves with a barrage of statements that include the word *should*. The "shoulds" are the demands that must be satisfied in order to transform the neurotic person into his idealized self—and his failure to live up to them leads to the slow, seeping growth of self-hate.

Reading *Neurosis and Human Growth* was an astonishing experience. Horney wrote about things I didn't know anyone else had noticed, let alone been able to explain. At moments, getting through it felt difficult and almost embarrassing; Horney hadn't even had to meet me to see me at my worst. She had grasped the feelings of superiority I tried to hide, even from myself, and also the appalling lack of confidence that was right beside it. She understood what I'd never been able to, which was how the two could coexist, how they were actually functions of one another. But it was the understanding, of course, that made the reading bearable. It was worth being flayed a little to get a wise take on old mysteries.

But it wasn't all flaying, either. Horney's ideas didn't just make intuitive sense to me; the way she talked about neurosis felt good, even hopeful, in a way that the chemical-imbalance theories never had. She thought, for one thing, that almost all people were neurotic to some degree, and that our society tended to make us so. While she didn't think that neurosis was healthy, she believed that struggling with it was a basic theme in human life. (As if to underscore the idea, she often illustrated her points with examples drawn from world literature.) I liked the way her theories seemed to imbue mental suffering with a meaning, and therefore a dignity, that had always been conspicuously absent from the discourse of faulty neurotransmitters. Thinking about having a chemical imbalance had always made me feel helpless, the victim of forces beyond my control. To my twenty-first-century ears, the word *neurosis* sounded strange and old-fashioned at first, maybe even subtly non-P.C. But the idea behind it soothed and heartened me, making me feel legible to myself and connected to other people in a way that nothing else had.

John never mentioned any specific psychological theories, but it was easy to map what we were doing onto the process of therapy as Karen Horney described it. He even pointed out how often the little word *should* popped into my statements about myself, and he tried to help me see past it. Letting go of "should" is scary. The demands that I uncovered felt like responsibility itself. I was terrified of relaxing them—I'd be slovenly, I'd never achieve anything at all!—but peeling them back, and peeling back the constant, low-grade sense of anger at and disappointment with myself that they entailed, allowed me to begin to take a different, deeper kind of possession of my life.

It is in the context of the idea of "shoulds" that I understand one of the moments from therapy that I remember most clearly. In the spring of my second year at Cornell, I went in, and I didn't know what to talk about. John had told me to pay attention to feelings, though, so I said, "I'm feeling grumpy." He asked me why, and I told him I was feeling grumpy because I didn't want to do any of my schoolwork. I had readings and deadlines, but I wasn't excited about them. I had developed a new, almost scary sensation that I could simply ignore my work, not do it for a while. As I was trying to explain this feeling, I got choked up. The emotion caught me completely by surprise. I had thought this would be sort of a throwaway session, one where I didn't have much to say. John asked me how I felt, and I said I felt really weird; I apologized and said I had no idea I'd cry about this. Then I sat there and wept for longer than I'd wept about anything in therapy up to that point. John asked me if I'd ever really allowed myself to feel this way before, and I said, no, I hadn't. He asked what would happen if I stopped doing my work, and I said probably nothing, for a while. It felt so wrong, so screwed up not to care, and I sat there crying and crying. I wrote in my journal later that I'd "broken the Kleenex barrier, or at least the record for number of Kleenex used." Later we talked about elementary school, and I said I remembered feeling like the puppet of adults who took my good performance in classes as a sign of obedience, and treated me like I was special, while inside I both loved this feeling and resented it and, eventually, myself. "It feels crummy to be a puppet," said John, and I nodded and smiled and grimaced and blew my nose. Later still, he told me that he was glad I was doing this stuff now, that it's so much better to do it at my age than at forty. I felt fanatically grateful for the suggestion that he had some idea what it was I was doing,

me back to a calmer, more cheerful place, and quickly. But as I continued in therapy, I saw more clearly that there were things I had needed for a long time, as much or more than I needed drugs. Antidepressants had gotten me moving, but they hadn't given me the sense of direction I craved. They had picked me up, but they hadn't made me more self-confident in any meaningful way. In fact, it began to impress me how much, once antidepressants had gotten me over the hump of whatever immediate misery I was dealing with, I had been able to go back and inscribe some of my old problems onto the drugs themselves. Not knowing what I wanted in the world, for example, had given me a fear of being influenced and changed, which translated handily into a fear that antidepressants would change me. Having a tendency to write off and doubt my own achievements anyway, I found in antidepressants a perfect reason for questioning whether the things I did were real, or whether I truly deserved credit for them. During the time I lived in Ithaca, I kept on using antidepressants, but over those two years it was therapy that made me feel better in ways I had never experienced before.

Critically, therapy taught me about the magic of cause and effect: that the things I do really affect the way I feel. I learned that emotional junk food—"shortcuts" to intimacy, or whatever kind of immaterial gratification you may be seeking—will make you feel as queasy and malnourished later as real junk food will. Emotional life is not unlike cooking or growing a plant: if you take your time and put in quality materials, chances are that you will get good stuff out in the end. It may be funny that I needed to do deliberate work to absorb this elementary lesson, but I did. In a way, antidepressants had long been giving me the opposite message: if you suffer for no reason, because there is simply a glitch in your brain, then it doesn't make much difference *what* you do. For me, antidepressants had promoted a kind of emotional illiteracy; they'd prevented me from asking or noticing the reasons I felt bad, or appreciating the effects of the world on me.

Most of all, therapy helped by making me see that some of the things I like most about myself and some of the things I like least stem from the same sources. Before I came to John, I was used to feeling two different ways. Sometimes I felt capable, well composed, on top of the world. Other times I felt abject and lost and horrible. Antidepressants had contributed to this tendency; one group of feelings meant "sick," the other, "well." John taught me to reexamine those assumptions, to think about the relationship of the bad to the good. Slowly I began to realize that some of the qualities I value about myself—that I feel things strongly, that I'm sensitive, that I care about doing well and about things being right, for myself and in the world—were precisely the things that made it possible for me to get cast down. But at the same time, these were the qualities that allowed me, on a good day, to be empathetic, warm, observant. A good friend, a hard worker. Some people find comfort in thinking about depression as a kind of disease, but for me, recognizing it as a potential nested deep inside me, intertwined with the traits that made me strong, made me hate my depression less, and made me hate myself less too. Depression is pretty hard to love, but I did learn to regard at least my tendency toward it with a little fondness and a little humor that, I like to think, took the edge off.

As I began to see myself as more nearly whole and seamless, another thing happened: I started to feel less alone. I had learned on that front porch in Portland, and many times over the years that followed, that I was far from the only person to take an antidepressant. But each time the knowledge had hit me and then receded like a wave. Maybe it was because having that kind of problem wasn't something I wanted to associate myself with. After all, the premise of biological psychiatry is that depressed feelings—no matter how many millions of other people have similar ones—are fundamentally abnormal, moods apart. But the longer I went on in therapy, the less unusual my problems began to seem, and the more I started to see other people in the multiple dimensions that I had begun to make out in myself. The true picture was so much more complicated, and more *interesting*, than any division into categories of sick and well: we were all collections of strengths and weaknesses, trying our imperfect best to get along in a difficult world. I remembered a line from Karen Horney that perfectly captured this change in perception. As the result of a successful analysis, she had written, a person may "experience himself for the first time as a being neither particularly wonderful nor despicable but as the struggling and often harassed human being which he really is"[5]—in other words, as a person among other people, subject to the same problems and limitations, but deserving of the same enjoyments and respect.

Feeling less unique made me able to talk to other people more openly, and listen better too; when I did, I realized as if for the first time how many of my friends and acquaintances also had problems with depression and anxiety, though it wasn't always apparent at first. Amelia referred to herself, half-jokingly, as "neuraesthenic"; Jules, who seemed so happy-go-lucky, took Zoloft; Louise had been on antidepressants before. I began to notice how many of these people also possessed a certain cluster of traits: they were sensitive, moody, empathetic, creative, funny, demanding of themselves, self-absorbed at times, but also capable of joy and a deep interest in the things that moved them. I started to wonder whether people like this tended to cluster in the places I'd been drawn to, like academia and the arts. Maybe being a little melancholic was an occupational hazard of being a certain type of person in the world, an annoyance but also a feature that could pull us toward each other. If that were true, then depression lost even more of its sting; it was a potential to be fought by any means necessary when it became acute, but not something that needed to be feared or rejected for any reason other than its simple awfulness in itself.

ONE DAY IN the spring of my second year of school, I lay in the grass in a small park in Ithaca and realized I would leave. It was May. The leaves were green and it was finally warm enough to lie on a blanket on the ground in only a long-sleeved shirt. My mind wandered over the past and peered into the future. I realized that leaving wasn't a hypothetical choice; it was something that I could really do. I felt the sensation of freedom that I remembered from my long drive in the country. As before, it felt both somber and light. It felt real. I turned my head and looked at the world through blades of grass. The sun was getting stronger; parents took long, smooth strides through the park while around them children ran, tripped, and fell. I knew there would be leave-of-absence forms, explanations, logistics, and probably doubts. I knew it, but I tried to leave that knowledge aside and just lie there in that moment, when the choice in front of me seemed terribly clear.

I ANNOUNCED MY intentions. Summer came, and then August. My friends threw a party for me at the dive bar downtown. People I hadn't expected to show up did show up. My friend Maria, who was an MFA student, had a custom T-shirt made that said A PAINTER AT CORNELL ♥S ME. I'm wearing it in all the pictures of me hugging and kissing friends and acquaintances at the Chanticleer that night. The day I left, friends gathered at my apartment to help me pack and load; I ordered everyone pizza. The chicken farmer, who had moved back to town and resumed his previous occupation as a graphic designer, came by to check the knots and cables on my car.

Let me mention one final lesson of and benefit from therapy. Over the two years that I saw John regularly, I became less afraid of strong feelings. I learned that powerful emotions and destructive emotions aren't the same thing. Destructive emotions felt cramped and conflicted, like a frantic frightened animal running around and around in a circle. Other emotions, even negative ones, didn't have this turbid quality; they hurt sometimes, but they didn't harm. I learned that there is a difference between simple sadness and depressed sadness. Unlike depressed sadness, simple sadness doesn't feel like it's going to destroy you. Simple sadness is like a benediction, a flag planted in the ground to mark the spot, a flag that means "this is gone now, but it was good."

It was simple sadness that I felt for John when I left him. To call it simple doesn't mean that it wasn't powerful. I will never forget walking down the long, cool, echoing hallway of the DeWitt Mall, away from John's office, on the last day. The feeling was so big. It almost didn't have any qualities other than its size and intensity. It wasn't good, and it wasn't bad. It just was, and it was so much. I stopped at the landing for a moment and steadied myself on the stone window ledge. It washed over me like a hurricane and I gave over to it completely and then it was gone, and I was still there, walking.

7 | FLIGHT OF THE DODO BIRD: EVALUATING THERAPY

enjoyed therapy immensely. I came away from each session feeling better, or at the very least, interestingly different, from the way I had going in. Over time I could sense myself growing. I developed new ways of seeing the world, and the new faculties allowed me to respond to life in ways that I'd never known possible.

But is psychotherapy more than a pleasant pastime for people who like to talk about feelings? When it comes to treating depression and other specific mental problems, do the "talking therapies" work?

There is quite a bit of evidence suggesting that they do. Though mental well-being is, much like mental illness, difficult to quantify, decades of studies of various kinds of talk-based psychotherapies all point to the basic conclusion that psychotherapy helps people.[1] Specifically, about three-quarters of patients who do talk therapy show improvement on some concrete measure:[2] diminished symptoms, greater length of time between episodes, or a subjective feeling that the problem has decreased.[3] Therapy has been shown to be particularly effective when the therapist is an expert practitioner with a sure grasp of his technique (a mental health specialist of any kind is better than a family doctor)[4] and when the therapist and the patient have a trusting relationship.[5] In fact, research shows that the two most critical factors determining the success of a psychotherapy in any given case are the quality of the patient's rapport with the therapist, and the patient's and therapist's trust in the framework being used. These positive expectations matter much more than the particular approach you might select. Psychodynamic therapy, cognitive-behavioral therapy, interpersonal therapy, family therapy: all can be effective. If you like your therapist and believe that her brand of therapy can help you, it probably will.[6]

The fact that a caring practitioner and a motivated patient are more important predictors of success than the actual theoretical underpinnings of the work they do was first discovered in 1936 by a psychologist named Saul Rosenzweig. Attempting to answer the seemingly straightforward question of what type of psychotherapy works best, Rosenzweig collected all the research available to him and arrived at his surprising conclusion—they all worked equally well. He called the phenomenon "the dodo bird effect," after a scene in *Alice in Wonderland* in which a dodo bird judges a foot race that has no start or finish line; contestants run around randomly, and the dodo bird ends the race by declaring, "Everyone has won, and all must have prizes!" Rosenzweig's work has been updated many times throughout the years, always with the same basic results.[7]

In the mid-1990s, the dodo bird effect got some real-life backup from a survey of 2,900 mental health service users conducted by *Consumer Reports*, the largest of its kind ever undertaken. Respondents who received psychotherapy rated their experiences with it subjectively: almost all reported that therapy had been a help to them, and that they'd made progress toward resolving the problems that brought them to treatment in the first place.[8] The type of therapy was not important, but the duration mattered; the longer the time people had stayed in therapy, the better their results.[9] *Consumer Reports* called the survey "convincing evidence that therapy can make an important difference,"[10] though critics have blasted the study for its selection bias, alleging that of course people who had a good experience would be motivated to crow about it.[11]

The dodo bird theory makes some people crazy. They want the efficacy of therapy to come down to something more standardizable than an ineffable bond between the therapist and the patient. Depending on your point of view, the dodo bird finding can be either a beautiful statement on the many possible paths to recovery, or a frustrating indication that all psychological techniques are equal parts mumbo jumbo, and that we may never satisfyingly separate placebo effects from real ones in this realm. Personally, the theory doesn't surprise or threaten me. Certainly, the desire to be able to quantify the effects of therapy makes sense. But after my work with John, the idea that the therapist-patient bond and a mutual allegiance to the project are of utmost importance seemed only natural—and to wish for a way to distinguish between the content of the work and its human qualities struck me as both understandable and almost obtusely beside the point.

The type of therapy John was practicing is what's known as "psychodynamic psychotherapy." It's a form that evolved out of psychoanalysis as it was developed by Freud; in turn, psychodynamic therapy forms the basis for many other talk therapies that are practiced today. The basic belief informing psychoanalysis, which also finds expression in all the therapies descending from it, was that much of our mental lives are subconscious—that we're all guided in our actions by motivations that remain partly secret to us.[12] The psychoanalyst's job was to use careful listening and interpretation to help bring the analysand's hidden conflicts and disowned feelings to her awareness. Making them available for conscious examination would allow the patient to begin the sometimes arduous process of personal change.

Psychodynamic therapy is less intensive than psychoanalysis, and more casual: patients are usually seen once or twice a week, rather than four or five times, and they sit face-to-face with the therapist instead of reclining on a couch. But it shares several of the tenets of analysis, including the idea that transference—the feelings of the patient for the analyst, and vice versa—is key to the treatment. The psychodynamic approach is based on the idea that people are formed by their personal histories, that those histories create patterns of relating to the self and other people, and that the resulting patterns can become the cause of suffering or maladaptation. When these patterns arise in the transference between the therapist and the patient, they can be noticed, studied, and worked on. Even the name "psychodynamic therapy" is a nod to the importance of these patterns. A "dynamic" is a structured, repeating unit of interaction and feeling, one tiny article in what the anthropologist T. M. Luhrmann called "the grammar of a particular person's emotions."[13]

Psychodynamic therapy also shares with analysis a belief in the importance of emotion in the therapeutic encounter. It's not enough that the therapist helps the patient *understand* her problems; for real change to take place, the patient must be made to *feel* them, right there in the consultation room.[14] (As Freud once explained in a letter to Jung, part of the importance of transference is that it gives therapy the emotional charge that makes it function: "Where it is lacking, the patient does not make the effort or does not listen."[15]) Finally, like analysts, psychodynamic therapists are expected to observe certain restrictions on their behavior. Therapists are not to give direct advice, not to share many personal details about themselves, and not to introduce the mutual obligations that characterize friendship.[16] Counterintuitively, the restrictions of this "asymmetrical" relationship allow for the development of the unique form of intimacy that is necessary for the work.

But psychodynamic therapy isn't the only or even, right now, the most popular talking therapy going. These days, that distinction belongs to cognitive-behavioral therapy, or CBT, a modality invented in the 1960s by an American psychiatrist named Aaron Beck.[17] CBT is a short-term therapy, often designed to be completed in just twelve sessions, and it is highly "manualized,"[18] meaning that it follows procedures that are standardized and written out in detail; the idea is that one practitioner should be able to deliver CBT pretty much the same way as any other. In treatment, the therapist and the patient work together to identify the patient's dysfunctional beliefs, or "cognitive distortions," and then they work on concrete techniques to substitute more accurate thoughts and adaptive behaviors, which the patient practices outside of the office.

Because it is highly manualized, CBT is easier to study than many other forms of talk therapy. Indeed, when Aaron Beck designed CBT he was partly motivated by the goal of creating a psychotherapy whose effects could be empirically measured and validated.[19] This has led to a bit of a catch-22 situation. CBT is widely hailed as the psychotherapy "most supported by research," but it's also far and away the therapy on which the most research is available: 90 percent of controlled clinical trials of talk therapies look at CBT.[20] Those clinical studies do show CBT to be effective, often nearly as effective as medication, at treating a host of psychological ailments, including depression. The claim that CBT is scientifically validated, while other talk-therapy modalities aren't, glosses over the fact that other kinds of therapy haven't been subjected to the same kinds of rigorous scrutiny. But it's a claim that holds great appeal for insurance companies, which appreciate the idea of a clinically supported therapy that can accomplish in a dozen sessions what other therapies claimed to be able to do in an open-ended year or two.

As it happens, I had some CBT back in college, during sophomore year, when I was living in a house with Jeff and three other roommates, taking Wellbutrin, and feeling in need of a psychic tune-up. The practitioner was a therapist at the college health center. He assigned me a book—*Feeling Good*, by David D. Burns, MD, one of the standard texts in the field—and we worked through it together. I completed the homework assignments that CBT is known for: I made lists of my negative thoughts, identified the cognitive distortions associated with them, and came up with new, nondistorted thoughts or actions to take their place. My roommates had a record player in the house that year, and a few crates of LPs that Jeff had imported from his parents' garage. We often sat up until late in the night, listening to records, drinking cheap beer, and talking. Once or twice the guy who lived next door in the duplex, and who had a small daughter, would bang on the wall for us to turn it down. Gradually I became preoccupied with the idea that even when he wasn't banging, the neighbor could hear our noise and that he was sitting over there, disgruntled, silently hating us. I dutifully recorded these thoughts in my homework, flagged them as a case of "jumping to conclusions" (one of the ten "cognitive distortions" discussed in the book; others include "all-or-nothing thinking," "disqualifying the positive," and "catastrophizing"[21]), and wrote down what I'd try to do instead: remind myself that I didn't *know* how he was feeling, and that if he cared to complain, he would.

For me, CBT was moderately helpful. I still remember some of those lessons, and I can still use them to push back against my own negative thoughts and deliver myself a quick jolt of perspective. But there was plenty I was searching for at the time that CBT didn't provide. Most of all, it didn't answer my craving for a sense of meaning. At the time I felt wrapped up in uncertainty about who I was and what I ought to do in life. The therapy I did later with John nudged me slowly toward the realization that while those are important questions, sometimes it's most productive not to ask them directly, but to look for little clues to the answers in the process of living itself. But CBT, with its relentless focus on a set list of distorted thought patterns, didn't even provide a way for me to get those larger questions onto the table. During my twelve sessions, I kept feeling an impulse to interrupt my therapist and say, "Okay, but could we talk for a minute about what's *really* on my mind?"

As a counterpoint, I've since spoken to a number of people who found CBT extremely useful. David, thirty-one, completed a course of CBT after an intractable depression forced him to take a break for a semester from college. David had had a little bit of insight-based therapy in the past, and he'd resented all the attempts to make him dredge through his past, pick apart his family, or locate the source of his problems in his childhood—he just wasn't interested. David liked CBT's focus on the present, its circumscribed nature, and its emphasis on specific results. The approach sounded right to him, and true to the dodo bird theory; CBT worked better than other things he'd tried.

Grace, thirty-four, received CBT in college and also found that it corresponded nicely with her sense of what her problem was. "Cognitive-behavioral therapy was really good," she said.

> It felt much more effective than just taking medication every day. I liked having assignments. The way it was explained to me, it totally made sense. Like there can be a moment in a situation where an insecurity that you have can cause it to spiral totally out of control. And it felt like, "I definitely do that." It's like when you're reading your horoscope and you say, "I'm such a Sagittarius." That's how I felt about CBT. It was just like, "How did you know?" So I liked having assignments and trying to catch myself in those moments. It felt like something I could use on a day-to-day basis.

My sense now is that CBT and psychodynamic therapy cover a lot of the same ground, but that psychodynamic therapy tills deeper. A psychodynamic approach would use your worries about your noise levels and your neighbor's displeasure as a jumping-off place to explore your personality structure: *Why do you care so much what your neighbor thinks of you?* the therapist might ask. *Where does your mind go when you're worrying about his disturbed peace and quiet? What else in your life does this situation remind you of?* In CBT, it doesn't matter so much why you jump to a given conclusion, just that you notice yourself doing it; in psychodynamic therapy, understanding *why* would be seen as essential to creating change. Which approach will work best for any given person probably depends on what kind of investigation appeals most. Are they more comfortable isolating and zooming in on the problem, or would they rather start by taking a slow, meandering walk to get the whole lay of the land?

Personally, I am an inveterate big-picture person, which made CBT's granular tendencies feel hampering. But it wasn't just that. The greater emphasis placed on the relationship between therapist and patient in psychodynamic therapy was something that I wanted and needed. A couple of months into our work, the thought occurred to me one day that John knew me better than anyone else ever had. An instant later, I reflected that that was absurd: I'd never even seen him outside of our two weekly hours in his office. But in a sense, it *was* true. The ritualized nature of our conversations allowed me to show and tell him things I'd never revealed to anyone else. In the grand scheme of things, these weren't remarkable revelations. But we all have sides of ourselves we'd prefer to hide, wishes and fears we go through life vaguely hoping that no one else can see. And though nobody claims to know exactly why interpersonally oriented therapies work, I think that the experience of being able to manifest all that you find most dubious about yourself to another person—a person who doesn't go screaming from the room but, actually, miraculously seems to see it all and care about you anyway—must have something to do with it. There is a standard line of jokes about therapy that have to do with people complaining that they feel pathetic paying someone good money just to listen to them, but the crazy truth is that inside of a good therapeutic relationship, it isn't just about money changing hands; the therapist's feeling for the patient is real. Over time, that capacity to care for and empathize with the patient is transferred, eventually becoming something the patient can do for herself. (Freud once wrote that in therapy, "Essentially, the cure is effected by love."[22]) When it works, it's a profound and mysterious, maybe even mystical, process. No wonder it bedevils those who dream of "evidence-based psychotherapies" as standardizable as the dose of a pill.

IT IS OFTEN said that psychotherapy in combination with medication is the best treatment for depression. These claims come from the many studies that have looked at medication and therapy (usually CBT), both alone and in combination, and compared with a placebo. The largest study of this kind with youth, the Treatment for Adolescents with Depression Study (TADS), sponsored by NIMH and completed in 2004, compared Prozac, CBT, and the two in combination against a placebo in a group of 439 youths aged twelve to seventeen who had moderate to severe depression. The study found that CBT and Prozac alone were each highly effective, while the combination provided a boost: at eighteen weeks of treatment, 85 percent of patients on combination therapy had responded, compared with 69 percent on Prozac alone and 65 percent on CBT alone. (At thirty-six weeks, the bump provided by combination therapy had decreased some, with 86 percent of the combination group responding, compared to 81 percent apiece for the Prozac group and the CBT group.)[23]

Besides being supported by data, combination therapy makes a certain kind of intuitive sense, particularly in cases of severe depression. Someone who's stuck deep in a rut of ruminative thoughts or lacks the energy for basic self-care is less likely to benefit from psychotherapy than somebody who has a bit of energy for the struggle. (Commenting on the inappropriateness of talk therapy to achieve "an immediate transformation of general mood," Andrew Solomon wrote, "When I hear of psychoanalysis being used to ameliorate depression, I think of someone standing on a sandbar and firing a machine gun at the incoming tide."[24]) Antidepressants, the reasoning goes, may be able to blast somebody out of an entrenched depression and put them in a place where they'll be able to properly do the work and absorb the benefits of therapy. Therapy, in turn, can help that person cope with symptoms that remain. It can make them better able to take care of themselves and recognize their triggers, so that they become less likely to get depressed again, or quicker to seek help when they do. And it can give them the skills to adjust to life as a healthy person, bestowing what my interviewee Mark called "the skill set to handle a nondepressed self." This learning/rehabilitation process might be especially important for people whose depression is long-standing and entrenched. Dan's story gives a good example of what people mean when they say that therapy and antidepressants together make the best medicine.

Dan was twenty-eight, but in person he gave the impression of someone a few years younger, just pulling his life together for the first time. He lived in Brooklyn, and if you passed him on the street, what you would see is a typical urban hipster: full beard, band T-shirt, visible tattoos. Though he is an assimilated New Yorker now, Dan was born and raised in a tiny rural community in Nebraska. "I knew everybody in the whole town," he told me. "It was all one culture, one type of person." He remembers it as a comfortable and unchallenging social world—maybe verging on

using antidepressants, particularly his fears that Paxil would dull his creative edge, while the therapist sat there, "just listening to what I said and writing notes, to determine what medication I needed to take."

After college, Dan moved around the country for a couple of years. He didn't have health insurance, so he stopped taking Paxil. It was only after going off medication, he said, that he fully realized what an impact it had been having on him. "It was a very sudden change I noticed," he said. The problems he'd had at the beginning of college had never completely gone away, but after graduation they quickly got worse. He also developed problems with anxiety that he'd never experienced before: "just things like feeling like I was going to have a heart attack, or not being able to ride in cars because I was afraid that I'd jump out." Over the next couple of years, he said, he tried to "psych myself out" of feeling that way, with mixed success.

In his mid-twenties, Dan settled in New York, where he landed a job working for a real estate developer. The money was good, but he still felt lost, and he was still experiencing symptoms. "It was the worst and best time of my life," he said, "because I was doing well professionally, but it was a dark period of my personal life. And I was depressed. I'd started going into these cycles every couple weeks where I'd be severely depressed for a while, and then not. I was drinking all the time and surrounding myself with my friends. When I wasn't with them, I was depressed. Even when I was around them I was depressed." Dan grew to loathe his job, and his anxiety problem returned. He couldn't sit still, so he'd slip out of the office and take walks, just wander the streets of Midtown for as long as he could get away with. "The anxiety thing had gotten progressively worse over the previous five or six years," he said. "I got to a point where I really couldn't deal with it anymore." Dan found a psychiatrist and began taking SSRIs again. But the first few kinds he tried didn't work, and when his anxiety and depression spun out of control, Dan ended up checking himself into the hospital. He stayed there for a few days, and started a new regimen of medications—adjusted over time, they now included a tricyclic antidepressant and a mood stabilizer. He was also assigned a therapist to work with after his release.

Dan has thrived since then. He told me that being in the hospital changed his point of view; for the first time, he began to think of depression as an illness to be treated, rather than a fate to be endured. The combination of medications he's on now is great, he said. He feels balanced in a way he never did on the antidepressant he took before. Comparing the way he feels today with the way he felt on Paxil in college, Dan said, "Now is completely different. Now I feel like this is the best feeling I've had in my life, ever. And I absolutely feel now that I cannot stop taking medication, ever, really."

But Dan doesn't think that medication is the whole story of why he feels substantially better this time. Even back in college, he told me, he believed that he was dealing with two orders of problem. One seemed more arbitrary to him, more chemical, while the other felt like it was related to the things that happened in his life. While medication helped with the first kind of depression, Dan said, therapy has been more effective at dealing with the second. "After I started taking Paxil I definitely thought that there was a chemical issue, that it was certainly helping a bit," he said. "The thing the Paxil helped me deal with was this overall feeling of depression, or like this really terrible mood out of nowhere. Let's say I'm walking down the sidewalk and I'm suddenly insanely depressed [for no reason]. I'm just walking someplace and I'm having these suicidal thoughts. That kind of went away when I was taking Paxil." And, he added, those feelings returned after he stopped taking medication. But even when he was on Paxil, "Certain events would still make me upset because I felt like I didn't know how to deal with those things. Just the normal social development that most people go through fairly early in life, I was trying to deal with when I was twenty years old." Even today, Dan says, medication takes away the "overwhelming or out-of-nowhere feeling of depression" that he believes is chemical, but it leaves the problems he thinks stem from his upbringing intact. And that, he said, is where his therapist comes in.

Dan told me he had been working with the same therapist since his release from the hospital; he described her as being "like a very confident, knowledgeable, wise friend." He said that therapy was most valuable to him as a kind of reality check—pointing out that long-standing depression, and even medications themselves, had left him understandably confused about what it is to feel normal. "I think when you're depressed," he said,

and especially when you're taking medication, a lot of times you're very confused about "Okay, how do I feel about this situation? Is this the way I'm supposed to feel about it? Or is the medication supposed to make me feel not that way? What am I supposed to be doing? Am I depressed? Am I not depressed? Is this normal for a person to feel?" Especially when I was back [on medication], I was like "Is it normal for me to feel this way?" I have a very good therapist who's very realistic and blunt, and she'll say, "That's totally normal," or "That's not."

Dan explained that his therapist had been helping him figure out the way different factors in his life affected him, things that the turbulence of his life before—between depression, anxiety, his drinking, and stress at work—had prevented him from noticing. For instance, he said, she made him appreciate how much his real estate job really was contributing to his unhappiness. "She convinced me that the job had a huge role in the way I was feeling overall," he said. "Whereas I had tried to justify a lot of the things that were happening to me in my mind by saying, 'I'm drinking,' or 'It's because I'm not good enough socially to cut it in that environment,' or 'My self-esteem is too low.'" She encouraged him to take his feelings seriously and leave that job for one that suits him better, and she convinced him to take a break from drinking. With the chemical aspect of his depression, the oppressive job, and the drinking habit gone, it was easier for Dan to observe what it was like to feel well, and to experiment with different ways of protecting his mood. "I can now say for certain that there are things that make me upset," he said. "Certain movies, certain books, certain music. And now I have the awareness to say, 'Maybe I shouldn't go there,' if I'm leaning toward that sort of mood."

Dan said he was also using therapy to work on his self-image. "Over the last ten years, when I was drinking and when I was depressed, I saw myself as this very unhappy, unfriendly person, this very moody type of character," he said. "And I would sometimes say that to people and they would completely disagree with me, like 'What are you *talking* about?' So over the years it's become more apparent to me that my self-perception is very off base." (It was hard for me, too, to imagine Dan as the brooding-misanthrope type. He was warm and unguarded, and made delightful company.) Dan said he was slowly dismantling his old identity and replacing it with a sense of himself that's more accurate. "When I was younger it was very much a self-esteem thing, physical issues, but now it's more about 'How do people see me as a person?'" he said. "Do people see the depression and the moodiness and this underlying anxiety, or do they not?" He recrossed his legs on the secondhand coffee table in his living room, where we were sitting. "And I'm starting to realize that people don't see that at all. But my therapist and I are still working on making me believe it."

Cumulatively, Dan refers to the changes he's gone through in therapy as the development of "self-awareness." Depression distorts, he said, and therapy has been of service by helping him get in touch with reality in a way that medication alone couldn't do. "Therapy plays a huge role in this self-awareness thing," he said. "I should give my therapist a lot of credit. It took someone with a completely neutral view of the situation to help me figure this stuff out."

AS I'M SURE you can tell by now, I am a big believer in therapy. I think that it offers a unique set of benefits that often make it a wise addition to medication, and that there are some problems for which it's an appropriate response on its own. Therapy teaches self-understanding and self-mastery in ways that medications do not. It makes people feel better about themselves and more in control of their lives in a global sense, while also diminishing specific symptoms. These benefits come at no physical risk. And unlike the effects of a pill, they last forever—actually deepening and strengthening as they're reinforced by life and time.

It's worrisome, then, to watch therapy's decline relative to antidepressants. Though evidence and anecdote suggest that the two work well together, Americans have become demonstrably more likely to reach for the medication and skip the therapy completely. A recent large-scale study reported that among antidepressant users in the U.S., the number also receiving therapy fell almost 40 percent from 1996 to 2005. A third of people taking antidepressants were getting therapy in the mid-1990s; a decade later, only 20 percent were.[25] Even though many experts recommend that antidepressants be used as a second-line treatment, to be tried only after psychotherapy is attempted and has failed, this sequencing is rarely carried out in practice. SSRIs are increasingly likely to be the sole remedy for an emotional problem.[26]

There are several factors at work besides consumers' wishes that encourage the increased use of medication as a first-line (and often stand-alone) treatment. One of those factors is health insurance. While patients sometimes state a preference for psychotherapy instead of or in addition to medications, weekly therapy sessions are undeniably expensive—and in recent decades, most health insurance companies have grown increasingly reluctant to cover their cost. Where benefits do exist, patient copayments for therapy sessions tend to be higher, sometimes much higher, than copayments for medication services, and the number of visits allowed per year is often restricted.[27] Coverage for SSRIs, by contrast, is usually unlimited.

These changes are a legacy of "managed care," the insurance model that became prevalent in the United States in the 1980s. Managed care is a cost-control strategy premised on the idea that the insurance company will pay for the least-expensive effective treatment for a given illness. In addition to a decreased willingness to pay for psychotherapy, managed care has been associated with a push to have general practitioners, rather than specialists, act as gatekeepers for care and provide more services themselves. These days, the majority of prescriptions for antidepressants are written not by psychiatrists but by general practitioners, who do not provide therapy or even a semblance of it. Managed care has pushed psychiatrists away from providing talk therapy, too, by reimbursing them at much higher rates for prescribing medication.[28] Timothy Dugan, a child and adolescent psychiatrist at Harvard's Cambridge Hospital, told me that insurance will pay him more for a twenty-minute "med check," where he adjusts a patient's medications and writes a fresh prescription, than it will for a fifty-minute hour of psychotherapy. He did a little back-of-the-envelope calculating and estimated that, at least as an MD who can do either, he can earn $450 in an hour (by doing three med checks), or $125 for giving an hour of therapy.

For psychiatrists, these financial incentives are understandably hard to resist. Many have shifted the emphasis of their practices away from therapy and toward medication; thanks to shorter and less-frequent appointments, psychiatrists who once managed fifty or sixty patients at once may now handle client loads of more than a thousand.[29] While psychiatrists used to provide psychotherapy along with medication, now prescriptions come from the doctor, and talk therapy, if it's wanted, from a different practitioner altogether. The situation leaves psychiatrists less able to monitor their patients' progress, because they see their patients less frequently and talk to them less extensively. It has also contributed to a shift in which psychotherapy, because it's generally no longer provided by medical doctors, has come to seem increasingly less like a medical service. The issue isn't quality—nonpsychiatrists can be excellent psychotherapists. But pushing therapy to the periphery of medicine strengthens the rationale for insurance companies not to fully cover it. Talk therapy joins the ranks of other "nice but not necessary" services, like acupuncture or massage, that can seem vaguely alternative and that consumers often expect to have to pay for themselves, while medical care for emotional problems becomes increasingly synonymous with pharmaceuticals.

Another factor that elevates medication and marginalizes talk therapy has to do with the way scientific research is funded. Academic careers in science and medicine are built on original, published research. Research is funded by grants, and grants are made by granting institutions; even researchers employed by universities are expected to finance their work with money from outside. (Indeed, it's a proven ability to nab funding that helps make academic job candidates in the sciences attractive to potential employers in the first place.) In psychiatry, the vast majority of grant money comes from pharmaceutical companies—which, unsurprisingly, are interested in funding work that highlights the clinical benefits of potential new products, not the merits of un-patentable talk treatments. "If you have a research career, by and large it's funded by drug companies' drug trials," Timothy Dugan explained to me. The upshot is clear: most of the research that's done in psychiatry is done on medications, and most of the people who've become influential in the field are people who are personally and professionally invested in the promise of psychopharmaceuticals, not talk.

The shift away from talk therapy is both reflected and

perpetuated in psychiatrists' medical education. I spoke to a young psychiatrist in New York City who told me that she feels lucky to be able to practice the way she wants—she provides talk therapy to most of her patients, in addition to medication—because there are enough people in the city who are willing and able to pay a premium for these services. She said she is disappointed that psychiatry has moved away from therapy. She thinks this happened because insurance has made therapy less lucrative; because psychiatry has been trying to legitimize itself as a "real" medical specialty, which means prescribing pills—the ethos is "We're real doctors, we don't do that touchy-feely thing anymore," she told me; and, she suspects, because prescribing drugs is less demanding. "It's much easier to write a prescription and hand it to someone than it is to really sit there and focus on them for 45 minutes," she said. Psychiatry has been deemphasizing therapy for so long, she continued, that the type of person who is drawn to the specialty is changing too; the field no longer necessarily attracts people who want to work closely and deeply with their patients' inner lives. "I think there are some people who are just uncomfortable being a therapist," she said. "And a lot of residency programs don't provide so much training. You're not trained to be a therapist, and you don't feel good in the role of a therapist, because that takes time too."

THE DECLINE IN access to therapy is a shame. The data support therapy as an effective treatment option, and they support the power of therapy when combined with medications. Therapy doesn't carry the risk of side effects. It helps people whom antidepressants don't help. And some patients prefer it to taking drugs. A number of the people I interviewed lent credence to the *Consumer*

Reports survey's contention that for many people, therapy can be a profoundly positive and lastingly helpful experience. I want to end with a few of their comments.

Isabel, age twenty-seven, of New York, took antidepressants all through high school and college, before quitting them just a couple of years ago. She'd had therapy on and off earlier in her life, but often at her parents' insistence; because she often didn't want to be there, she said, she didn't get much from the experience. Isabel looked for a therapist on her own in her early twenties, when she was in a graduate program for fine arts and feeling unhappy about school and unsure of her direction. She described to me how good it felt to find somebody she clicked with.

One therapist that I had when I was in high school was helpful up to a point, and then she just wanted to talk about my relationship with my father a lot. And I was like, "I don't want to talk about that. I don't think that's really very relevant." But she was very pushy, and it felt like it was her agenda rather than my agenda.

Then I saw one when I first got to New York, and I *loved* her so much. She was great because she was really focused on the events of my actual life. We talked about underlying things, but she was the first one who felt like I was capable of changing things in my life which would then make me feel better. That was very helpful.

I was like, "I don't like painting grad school, it feels silly." And she said, "Maybe you would like to do something like advertising." And I was like, "No one has ever said anything like that to me before." She said maybe part of the reason you don't want to leave school is because your mother likes art and wants to be an artist, and I was like, "Yeah, I see *that* connection."

Therapy can also help the sizable portion of people who don't get substantial relief from antidepressants. (One major study concluded that around 30 percent of people who try antidepressants ultimately find them ineffective; critics contend that the real figure might be much higher.[30]) Now twenty-five and living on the East Coast, Elizabeth was the child of diplomats, and grew up all over the world. Elizabeth got depressed in middle school, and the embassy psychiatrist prescribed antidepressants to her when she was fifteen. She has taken them ever since, sometimes switching brands or dosages, looking for a stronger effect, but she's never felt that medications gave her more than minor benefits. Elizabeth started doing therapy for the first time after she finished college, and she said that it's helped her to a view on her situation that feels more accurate than the idea of simply having a chemical imbalance. In therapy she started to look at the role she'd played in her family, where she weathered conflict by "trying to be really good all the time, and never hurt anybody else's feelings," patterns she now believes had a lot to do with the problems that emerged when she was a teenager. Therapy helped her understand how her behavior developed over time and how it has contributed to the way she feels, and that understanding has brought her a new kind of relief.

I eventually have started to come around to the realization that my reaction to my situation when I was a kid didn't occur because there was something wrong with me. It was because I was actually reacting like a normal person. I actually had plenty of things to be angry about, and there were plenty of good reasons why I repressed it.

Honestly I was never sure whether the antidepressants were working. Partly because I didn't know what "working" would entail. And it's only more recently when I've been in therapy and have been working on dealing with my anger that I've started to feel a lot better. And have actually sort of started to understand what that might mean.

Dana, from Boulder, began going to therapy around age ten, when her parents were divorcing. She started taking Prozac when she was fifteen, and continued both talk therapy and medication through the end of high school. Now thirty-one, she is finishing up a doctoral program in psychology—so moved was she by her experiences in therapy as a teenager that she decided to become a therapist herself. Dana told me that when she looks back on her high school years, it's hard to separate the influence of the two approaches. But when she thinks about it, she believes that for her, the therapy was the more essential experience. "If I had not had treatment for depression (therapy and/or medication), I am sure my life would have been different," she explained in an e-mail. "I'm inclined to attribute the majority of the helpful influence to my therapy, which has been introspective, relational, supportive, reassuring, challenging, enriching, and really valuable to me." In our conversation, she summed it up like this:

I think that, in theory, I could have made it through my adolescence without antidepressants, and found myself in much the same place I am now. I could not have made it through my adolescence without psychotherapy. I can't imagine just having said to my parents, "I feel depressed, and sometimes I want to kill myself," and having them take me to a shrink who sat with me for twenty minutes, and gave me pills, and sent me on my way. I just can't even conceive of that experience.

Nathan, also thirty-one, lives in Kentucky. He told me that his life was finally beginning to feel calm and stable after major turbulence throughout his twenties. In college, Nathan developed problems with substance abuse and drinking, to the extent that he was expelled from school. He moved to a major city, where he continued drinking heavily and using cocaine. He got into legal trouble and did lots of what in therapy-speak is called "acting out": he got into fights, had screaming matches with his girlfriend, and once drunkenly slammed a door and severed a part his own finger. In college, he began to experience manic episodes, and they continued afterwards. He tried various antipsychotics, including Seroquel and Risperdal, and had terribly mixed experiences with them; they helped somewhat but also caused "horrible physical and cognitive side effects." Through it all, Nathan wanted to find someone he could talk to. "I could find plenty of prescribing doctors, but to find anybody who would talk to me was impossible," he said. He saw one psychiatrist he hated so much he didn't want to return, and he stopped taking his medication. "I didn't like this doctor," he said. "I felt like he spent more time telling me about his own children and his words of wisdom for them than about me; he didn't really want to find out too much about me. And that's one reason why I quit taking those drugs, was that I never wanted to go back to see him to refill the prescriptions."

Nathan bounced around the country for a while, in and out of schools and relationships—still, by his own admission, abusing drugs and alcohol. Around the holidays in 2006, he ended a serious relationship with a woman who had been scared away by his mental problems. He was twenty-five, and he decided it was time for a big change.

> Around Christmastime 2006, I moved back home, and
> around the end of February, I found a therapist. I told him I
> wasn't going to go on any medication, that I wasn't drinking,
> I'd quit smoking cigarettes, I was training to run a marathon
> in three months, and I just wanted to talk to the guy. He was
> a young man. I really liked him. He was a great listener. He
> listened enough that I felt comfortable with him enough that
> I basically just started saying out loud things that I could
> then puzzle through myself. I talked to him for about three
> months, and at the end of the three months I felt, honestly,
> like the whole ordeal was done.

I asked Nathan what he thought therapy had done for him. He told me it had helped him to process a lot of what had been bothering him in his earlier twenties, and to deal with the problem of his own expectations for himself. He had wanted to be an academic, but his mania and his drug use had forced him to lay those dreams aside. Therapy helped him adjust to the loss of the life he'd imagined and focus on his daily reality. "I think we spend a lot of time up until somebody says 'Okay, this is your life, do what you want with it,' creating illusions about what that's going to be like, and what you can do," he explained. "Other people had expectations for me, but really most of them were expectations I'd built for myself. And to start to see those unravel is a painful thing."

He continued:

Here's the difference between me now and me then. Me now realizes that grief and pain are not endless, you know? And they're not useless. I'm not afraid of pain so much that I need to go tell somebody, "I think I'm about to hurt, and I'm really scared; is there any way you can make me not hurt?" I do feel much more confident in myself for having—my therapist basically gave me the courage to sit with that pain for as long as it takes before you can understand it and it goes away.

For a while I even wanted to be a therapist, because I felt so strongly about talk and the power of talking. I still feel very strongly about it.

8 | QUITTING

The autumn after I moved back to New York, I stopped taking my Zoloft. I didn't make any grand pronouncements to myself or anyone else about going it alone. I just decided, quietly, to take a little bit less, and a little bit less, and then less still. A hundred milligrams a day became 75, then 50, then 25—one buttermilk-yellow capsule, to a half, to a quarter, to the point where tiny slivers of pill turned to dust between my fingertips, and I couldn't swallow a smaller dose. Tapering down took months, but it was privately thrilling: the feeling of wading one, two, three steps farther out from shore, feeling the lake bottom bounce away underfoot, and finally, floating free.

In hindsight, it surprises me that stopping should have felt so dramatic. But it did. By that point, in 2006, I had been taking antidepressants for nine years, punctuated by only a few short breaks. And like a lot of people who use antidepressants for a long time, I had developed a side effect not printed on the label: a fear of living without them.

Partly, the sense of adventure was an indication of how mysterious and even off-limits the topic of quitting antidepressants can be. For a long time it had seemed remarkable to me how little people talked about it; in a culture that couldn't shut up about antidepressants—whether you should go on them, how you would know—discussion of the corollary question seemed strangely absent. There were no helpful magazine articles about judging whether it was time to chuck your Prozac, or how to do it the smart way. More surprisingly, no doctor I had seen had ever broached the issue, either to warn me that I should never stop, or to tell me when I might expect to or how to approach the decision. The few times when I tried to bring it up, the line of questioning didn't feel especially welcome, and the present-focused replies—*This seems to be working now; why don't you just stay on it?*—felt as though they concealed the lack of a larger answer.

In fact, most of the advice I'd ever heard about getting off of medication was practical, not "whether" but "how." I had read that weaning oneself off slowly was preferable to quitting cold turkey. Tapering was supposed to prevent "discontinuation syndrome," stories of which had begun to surface in the news media and the urban-legend network by the mid-2000s. It seemed that some people, getting off some antidepressants—notably the SNRI Effexor, but also the SSRI Paxil, among others—experienced a host of unpleasant side effects that could last for weeks or months, including the frighteningly-named "brain zaps," which were often likened to the feeling of a sharp electrical shock inside one's head. I had even heard it whispered in a few places that discontinuation syndrome could involve emotional symptoms as well as physical ones, making it possible that some number of people who went off their medication and then had a relapse quickly weren't actually experiencing "true" depression, but a form of drug withdrawal instead. I had no way of judging these claims, which felt a bit like early-1970s hippie paranoia to me, but they provide an example of how fraught the whole topic of quitting had come to feel. That the stories existed suggested that some people were doing it. But the tales often had the same vigilante tone, a sense of confused people feeling the need to take matters into their own hands.

In a way, the lack of free-floating official guidance made sense. Depression can be dangerous, and perhaps for that reason, doctors and other experts are loath to put forth one-size-fits-all proclamations about quitting. Many doctors, and some laypeople too, seem to believe that once started, antidepressant therapy should go on more or less forever—and in some cases that may be absolutely right. There is still a little touchiness around the fact that depression was and is a stigmatized illness; some may feel that to talk about quitting medication is to question the seriousness of the disease, or to confront suffering people with the damning and probably incorrect idea that they *could* be okay on their own, if only they would *try harder*. That reasoning is understandable. But given that millions and millions of people start using antidepressants, for a great variety of reasons, it seems equally outrageous to assume that everyone ought to stay on their medications indefinitely, or that collectively skirting the issue is the approach likely to lead to the best and safest outcome for all.

As it turns out, there are some guidelines regarding how long people should stay on antidepressants, but I had to do a little journalistic sleuthing to find them. One psychiatrist I talked to told me that as a rule of thumb, an adolescent with a first episode of depression should be maintained on an antidepressant for about six months following a full remission of symptoms; after that, the dosage could be brought down slowly and the patient monitored for signs of a recurrence. Subsequent episodes, he said, should be dealt with more aggressively, with antidepressant therapy maintained for longer; after a third episode, continuous maintenance on an antidepressant was advisable.

But in practice, those guidelines are far from universally applied. My own experience was more like that of Alexa, who in talking about antidepressants spoke offhandedly of "the way they're prescribed to sort of never end," or Dana, who said that one of her motivations for quitting antidepressants was the fact that "nobody was having a conversation with me about ever going off them, and that seemed odd." It seems safe to say that many doctors feel more comfortable getting people started on antidepressants than coaching them off. If the patient seems to be doing fine on medication, the feeling seems to be that it's fine to keep them there. And in a world where patients who take psychiatric drugs are often seen in fifteen-minute increments that may fall months apart from one another, it's easy to grasp why physicians might feel reluctant to rock the boat.

In the absence of clear advice about how long a course of antidepressant treatment should last, many people adopt a self-guided version of the pattern that the psychiatrist described to me. They take medication, stabilize on it, feel better for a certain period of time, and then experiment with taking themselves off.

That's certainly what I was doing. To date, I had quit antidepressants three times—the summer after my freshman year in college, at nineteen; the summer before graduate school, at twenty-two; and finally at twenty-six, not six months before returning to New York. I had been living temporarily in California, first doing a magazine internship and then looking for work. While I hadn't actually stopped taking Zoloft when I was living in Ithaca, I had gotten newly curious about it. I wondered whether the things I'd learned in therapy might make a difference. Was it possible that I'd become better at knowing, and meeting, my own needs in a way that could shift my relationship with medication? I didn't mean to quit just when I did, but with that question in the back of my mind, I let two events in California make the decision for me: I fell in love. And I ran out of prescription refills.

It was not a success. As with the other times I'd stopped, I felt fine for a few months, but toward the end of my time in the Bay Area, as the structures that had been giving my life shape fell away one by one, I drifted into a state of near-constant anxiety that left me exhausted and, eventually, practically galloping toward the office of a San Francisco psychiatrist. By the time I arrived in New York a few months later, I felt calmer but still bruised, like a vase that's been glued back together, serviceable but still shiny along the seams.

Some people would have called me foolhardy for trying again, or masochistic, or even ungrateful. At moments I wondered whether I was one or all of these. Still, I couldn't seem to resist trying again. I had my general reasons—I'd never wanted to stay on antidepressants forever—and my particular ones: coming to New York and starting a new job meant starting over again, and I wanted to be sure I knew how this new life was making me feel. It felt as though, after some delay, I was beginning to build the foundations of my adult life, and if something about that life was making me uncomfortable, I wanted to know it. Finally, I wanted to quit antidepressants simply because I believed that I'd feel a sense of achievement if I was able to live without them.

That belief had been with me for a long time. It felt problematic and un-P.C., but it was also stubborn. I knew that you weren't supposed to care if you used medications or not, that you weren't supposed to *root*. That you were meant to take them if you needed them and be okay with it.

But I couldn't help it. I wanted to stop if I could. And I had beliefs about why this time might be different. For the first time in years, I had moved to a city that I didn't have any immediate plans to leave. (I added it up and realized that I'd changed addresses twelve times since the end of college.) I had a full-time job, a regular schedule, and a roommate who was also a good friend. There were no big changes looming. All the previous times I'd quit, I realized, I'd done it before a major transition, and I wanted to test my theory that timing might have accounted for some or all of the failure. Finally, I had my new attitude. I was taking it slowly, almost comically slowly. I told myself that this was just an experiment. If I started to feel bad, I would go back up on the dosage—and it wouldn't be an all-time thing, just a hint that now wasn't the right moment. It didn't have to succeed. But I was also hoping, quietly hoping, that it would.

WITH GUIDANCE OR without, rashly or at a snail's pace, people do discontinue antidepressants, of course. During interviews for this book, I talked to ten people who described stopping antidepressants after spending a significant amount of time on them. They named a few major reasons for their decisions. Some felt that medication never worked well for them; they belonged to the 30 percent or more of people who either don't obtain significant relief from antidepressants, or develop side effects so intolerable that they can't continue. Some people, like Dana, cited the fear of unforeseen physical consequences of using antidepressants long-term as a major factor. At twenty-nine, Dana had been on Wellbutrin for about eight years continuously, and on other anti-depressants on and off for another seven years before that. "I was having some concerns about long-term effects," she said, "like a little bit of anxiety about what are these pills maybe doing to my brain in a long-term way." Also, she added,

> I was growing increasingly dubious about my need to be medicated in such a consistent manner. I didn't want to take them if I didn't need them. And I knew that I wouldn't ever know if I needed them if I didn't try to kind of set myself up for success by being thoughtful about it, and come off them, and see. —*Dana, age thirty-one*

Dana wasn't the only person who mentioned the fear of possible physical or psychological effects of staying on antidepressants for years. Are these worries founded? It's an interesting question. The SSRIs have been around for a quarter century now, and reports of serious cognitive or physical effects from extended use have yet to emerge. At the same time, no truly long-term studies have examined either the effectiveness of antidepressants beyond a few years, or systematically tested for long-term side effects. This lack of research largely reflects the fact that most studies of pharmaceuticals are driven by the FDA approval process, which requires that new drugs be shown to be clinically effective and not acutely toxic for a finite period of time, often in the range of weeks or months; there's no regulation that would require drug makers to test for side effects emerging years later. "Most of the data suggest that the adverse effects that happen with antidepressants happen relatively soon," said David Kupfer, a research psychiatrist at the University of Pittsburgh, who added that there is no evidence of harm from lengthy use of SSRIs. Still, questions like "Does this medication change my brain in a permanent way?" are questions that we don't yet have the definitive knowledge to answer.

Dana decided that her worry about long-term effects, coupled with her sense that antidepressants might never have been absolutely necessary for her, made it worthwhile to experiment with stopping. She didn't quit under a doctor's guidance, but she recalls trying to set herself up for success as methodically as possible. In college, she said, she had gone on and off her medication "on whims," and these discontinuations had often led to new depressive episodes and new prescriptions. This time she deliberately tried to stop at a point when her life felt stable. She was in her late twenties and wrapping up her second year of graduate school. "The year before had been pretty arduous, and kind of anxiety provoking, and tearful, but my second year had been a really great year, a bolstering and confidence-building year," she said.

> And I remember thinking, "Here I am in a pretty good place, feeling good about the path I am on, and feeling confident and stable about various aspects of my life." It felt like a safe time to experiment and get a clearer read on whether I could handle it.
>
> I was aware. I told my parents in advance. I told my boyfriend. And I also told myself that if this doesn't work and I have to go back on them, that's okay. This is not, like, the

test of a lifetime. If it doesn't work for me, and I need these again, I feel okay about that.

Was it hard to get off?

No. It felt, actually—I really had no effects. Over the course of about three weeks or a month, I weaned myself. I don't recall any negative effects at all.   —*Dana, age thirty-one*

Other people have motives for quitting that seem more intimate. They simply feel, for reasons they can't always articulate, that they'd prefer to get by without medication if they can. Meghan, twenty-five, described quitting antidepressants as a way of telling a different story about herself—and at the same time, she said, adopting a different story about herself was a way of moving beyond antidepressants. Her experience shows that just as starting antidepressants can be a process that takes place on two levels, combining the literal activity of taking medication with intangible revisions to one's sense of self, stopping medication can involve the same in reverse.

Meghan had found the idea of antidepressants off-putting from the start. In high school, she had struggled on and off with depression—"It wasn't always debilitating," she said—and during her junior year of college, she sought counseling through her school's mental health service. After a few months of sessions, her counselor suggested that Meghan be evaluated for medication. "She said, 'For someone who's as seriously depressed as you, it can be a good decision,'" Meghan remembered. "I was dumbfounded. I was like, 'I am seriously depressed?' The whole idea shocked me. But I'd really developed a rapport with this woman, I trusted her opinion, and nothing else seemed to be working."

Meghan's counselor referred her to a university psychiatrist. The appointment, Meghan remembered, lasted about half an hour. "The psychiatrist said 'You know, there's depression in your family, this is clearly genetic, you were born with this deficiency, and you're going to need to take these for the rest of your life,'" Meghan recalled.

> She didn't know me. But that was just her view of depression, and how to fix it. She thought that this was the way to go. And so I just had this idea like okay, well, if I want not to be depressed for the rest of my life, I guess I do have this deficiency, and I'm going to have to take a pill in order to fix that. So I was prescribed 20 milligrams of Prozac. Which, I went back after a month [for a follow-up] and I was like, "SOMETIMES, I WANT TO JUST BREAK THINGS OUT OF *LOVE*!" And she was like "Okay, well, maybe this is too high of a dose."

The psychiatrist reduced the dose, and Meghan stayed on Prozac through the end of college. She said that it made a favorable difference, but she never warmed up to the idea of taking pills for her mood. On the other hand, what the psychiatrist had told Meghan about needing Prozac forever stuck with her. Meghan used the words *story line* several times in our interview. She told me that the story given to her by the school psychiatrist intimidated her. "There were a couple of times that I decided I wanted to go off Prozac" during college, Meghan explained, "but every time I did, I would start freaking out, and that whole story line of what [the psychiatrist] told me would come back, and I would be like, 'I need this, I actually have to take this, you can't just go off it or you're not going to be able to function,' so then I would get back on."

Ultimately, Meghan said, receiving a new "story line" about herself from a different doctor was a critical factor that enabled her to stop. After she graduated from college, Meghan moved to a new city with friends. There, about three years after she began taking Prozac, "I ran out of medication at the turn of the year, and I tracked down a psychiatrist and was like, 'I really need a prescription.' He said okay, so I made an appointment." She went on:

So I go and see him, and give him my history. I tell him what the psychiatrist said to me, and my relationship with medication, and he's like, "Okay, Meghan. That is something that a lot of medical doctors believe. That you need this. But a lot of studies show that there are other things that can stimulate the same areas of the brain that medication does, and that one of the most effective uses of medication is in short bursts, around seven months, and that there are all these other things you can do, including effective therapy, and you really don't have to be on them forever."

And I was like, "Oh! Well, that's great news! Okay." And just him *telling* me that made me relate to the medication in a different way. I was like, "Oh, *right*. There are other things that can make you happy. It doesn't have to come from a pill." And just having this new story line, after a few months—I saw him for a little while but he was expensive—so I didn't stay in therapy, but it was enough to make me realize, okay.

With the new doctor's blessing, Megan went off Prozac. She remembers adopting a one-day-at-a-time approach to her moods, and especially making an effort not to see occasional bad days as confirmations of a story about needing medication forever. "The new story I told myself was 'Okay, well, today I'm going to feel sad, and that's okay, you can handle this; tomorrow you probably won't feel as sad, and that's great, you can handle that,'" she said. "And just that new story line helped me, and I haven't been on it since."

A surprising number of people described quitting antidepressants *during* a time of crisis. These decisions usually weren't premeditated, but happened on the spur of the moment. The people who made them acknowledged that stopping impulsively wasn't necessarily wise, but they spoke of feeling a need to make a big gesture—to assert control over something at a point when nothing else in life seemed to be going as planned.

Alexa, who had taken antidepressants since the time she was thirteen, remembered quitting abruptly at the end of her junior year in college. She had been having an intensely rough semester. "I got to a point where I was probably the most depressed I'd ever been," she said, "like just crying to the point where I was bursting blood vessels under my eyes for no reason."

This was while I was on a cocktail of MAO inhibitors and SSRIs and whatever the other one is, Wellbutrin. So I was on everything. And I was cleaning out my room from my junior year, and I was just like, "I'm going to throw them away and see what happens." That's the wrong way to go off them, of course; you're supposed to wean yourself off. But I was like, if I don't do this dramatically, it won't feel like I'm making a decision. And that's definitely the wrong way to do it. But I didn't have any bad effects. I basically didn't feel like anything happened except I stopped crying. I definitely felt a little numb for a few months. But this is from someone who used to have to raise her hand in class in college to [be excused to] go cry.   —*Alexa, age twenty-three*

A few months after stopping, Alexa said, "I kind of felt the same way that I had felt on the drugs. I mean, still having trouble. Still crying a little bit more than normal people." But it was nothing she couldn't handle, she explained. After many years on them, Alexa was fascinated to find that she seemed to be all right without medication. She even associated stopping with a kind of delayed adolescence. "I definitely felt freer," she said, adding that she began to explore sides of herself that she never had before. "Just really simple stuff, like I started wearing dresses. I dated the first boy I had dated in college my senior year," she said. "I was definitely more confident. I think most of my friends were like, 'Who is this new person?'"

Alexa described quitting antidepressants as an experiment, one that she would abandon if she ever felt like she needed to. (She told me that she had kept her last prescription in her wallet until long after graduation, just in case she ever wanted to fill it.) By the time we talked, though, it had been five years since she'd stopped using medication, and she said that she still preferred life without it. "I think I mainly went off them because I was just really curious what the hell is it going to feel like," she said. "And then I think I just liked it—I liked it more."

Abby was another person who quit at a time when things were at their absolute worst. Abby was twenty-seven when we met, tall and striking-looking, with dark eyes and glossy hair. She had a confident, assertive manner, and it surprised me when she started talking about her childhood, describing a pattern of abuse and neglect that had made her an outcast at school. "For me, it was always very social," she said. "I think depression is a disease the way poverty is a disease." Abby had been on various combinations of medications for most of the time since she was fourteen. However—perhaps unsurprisingly given the way she understood the nature of her problem ("I can pinpoint exactly why and how I feel the way I feel, and it doesn't have to do with necessarily my serotonin level, you know?")—she'd never found medication to be remarkably effective. Even so, I was startled and a little bit worried when she told me how she had stopped taking antidepressants, almost a year before we talked:

> I'd put myself into a horrible situation with a horrible man, a terrible job that I was not happy in, and I was not doing well. I was completely miserable, the winter was there, and it was a really, really low point. I realized that it was an abusive relationship. So, yeah, I decided that obviously this wasn't working, because I was putting myself in this position. I was at the bottom. And I swear, I told myself, at this point, I was super depressed, I was smoking weed all the time. And I had it in my head that I had AIDS. And then, yeah, I stopped taking antidepressants. I think it might have been a suicidal type of thing too. But what happened was I stopped taking the antidepressants, and then I purposefully lifted myself out of the situation.
>
> I called movers. I quit work. I broke my lease, I lost my deposit. All my furniture, I put in my parents' basement. My

friend was going overseas. I said, "Can I stay in your apartment, in Manhattan?" And there I was. No job, no boyfriend, nothing. And then I started my life all over again.

I'm not saying that all of a sudden everything was like rosy. Shit, no. But at least I did feel like I was closing the book on something. —*Abby, age twenty-seven*

In the months since then, Abby told me, she had moved six times, most recently to an apartment where she could stay for at least a year. She was working on a career realignment, into a related field she thought would suit her better. She told me that life still felt hard. While she was glad that she stopped antidepressants when she did, she said she had been thinking actively about getting back on them. Just the week before, she had gone to a psychiatrist and gotten a prescription for Wellbutrin, which was sitting in a bottle on her desk at home while she considered what she wanted to do.

WHETHER THEY DID so rashly or deliberately, almost everyone who quit described adopting new behaviors and new attitudes to help them manage life without medication. I had noticed myself doing the same thing. I was getting off Zoloft at the same time as I was settling into life in New York, and I found that I was establishing my routines in my new home with a care and a deliberateness that felt different to me. The noise and speed and off-the-rails liveliness of New York appealed to me as much as they ever had, but I also realized that I was paying new attention to carving out times and places to feel calm. I painted my new bedroom a warm shade of cocoa brown that made me feel cozy, and put up fluttering white curtains. While I was in graduate school, cooking had become a favorite ritual, something I found relaxing and nourishing in a way beyond just the literal, and I tried to keep the practice up in our tiny Brooklyn kitchen. On weekdays I packed vegetable lunches and, weather permitting, ate them over a book in the small park near the office of the magazine where I worked. I enjoyed the feeling of being able to take good care of myself.

As the Zoloft dosage came down and then down further, I did notice myself feeling a little bit different. It wasn't always marked. Most of the time I felt fine. But often, the anxieties that I already had would rise up a little, become sharper. I felt more emotional in all directions; I caught myself welling up more often on the morning subway train because something in the newspaper I was reading seemed moving, hit me right on the spot. It wasn't all bad. I liked having an intensity. It felt like a kind of return to something I'd forgotten. Every now and then I'd spot another red-eyed rider on the train, or pass someone walking the other way down the street, talking on a cell phone and crying. New York was amazing. People lived their lives out in the open, but the cumulative effect was so mysterious.

In exchange for these new sensitivities, perhaps, I found myself placing more importance on things like getting enough sleep, going home when I was through feeling social, running in the park. I made a conscious effort not to overburden myself or my schedule with commitments. In my journal, I wrote that I felt like a tightrope walker performing the same old routines, without a net this time. The simplest things felt a little more exciting, and I went around with a new consciousness that it was important to be careful. I had to be nice to myself; no one and nothing else was going to do it for me.

The people I interviewed also reported taking on new activities and having new feelings about old ones. Often they did this consciously, out of a sense that they could try to make up for the effects of medication with modified habits. Many said that exercise had become vital to them, and that it made a difference: Shannon did yoga; Isabel and Abby signed up for gym memberships. "Exercise has helped me a lot," said David. "This summer I've been running, and it's been amazing. I don't know what I'm going to do when winter comes." Quite a few people had used trial and error to arrive at a belief about what kinds of changes made the biggest difference for them. Shannon was trying to eat fewer processed foods, and Alexa said that she'd moved getting enough sleep to the top of her list of priorities. "I have to be really strict about sleep," she said.

> If I don't get enough sleep, I just start crying all the time. So what I do is I just go to bed early. If I'm out with my friends and it's midnight, I'm terrified, because I'm thinking, I'm going to get to sleep when it's 2:00 A.M. So, needless to say, [I've started to prioritize sleep over my] social life, because it makes me happier. And the two hours that I'm at that bar with my friends, that they're at for eight hours, are going to be better.
>
> And that was a big resistant thing, the sleep thing, at first. Most of my friends, even the very supportive, understanding ones, are like "Really? You're really going to bed now?" But that's just what I need to do.   —*Alexa, age twenty-three*

As it turns out, there is at least some scientific evidence for the influence on mood of changes in all these realms—exercise, sleep, and diet. A number of studies performed over the years suggest that exercise can have a therapeutic effect on depression; the benefits of two to four months of a sustained exercise program can be comparable to the benefits achieved by antidepressants. More vigorous exercise is correlated with greater relief. Moreover, there's evidence that exercise may have a preventive effect, making people who exercise regularly less likely to get depressed in the first place.[1] Sleep disturbances have been linked with depression too. While insomnia or oversleeping can be effects of depression, there's evidence that the direction of causality can also go the other way,[2] and that maintaining an erratic sleep schedule and habitually undersleeping can lead to disordered moods.[3] As for diet, though there is an avalanche of studies that have looked at the effect of single foods or nutrients on depression, the study I find most compelling (and, like many compelling studies, commonsensical) is one that tracked thousands of London office workers for years and found that, after adjusting for other factors, a "whole food" dietary pattern emphasizing vegetables, whole grains, fruits, and fish correlated with a lower risk of depression than a "processed food" dietary pattern.[4]

Not all of the interventions people mentioned were tangible. Meghan, Grace, and Shannon talked about the importance of community. "So much of depression is feeling isolated, and not being able to depend on anyone," said Meghan. She said that one of her theories about why she was able to stop using medication is that while she was on it, she was able to build up an excellent and supportive network of friends. "Through being on medication and being more happy and confident, I developed a lot of really good friendships. And I think that having a community helped me stay off medication ultimately. Just sort of not feeling like a total freak when I was having a hard time. Like my friends still loved me, and I'm just a person, and I'm having a hard time and that's okay." Alexa spoke about community in a slightly different way—she said that after quitting, she needed to regulate who she was spending time with and monitor what kind of effect they were having on her. "I had some very intense friendships and I was like, 'I'm not going to be friends with you anymore, because I can't handle it.' These were people who were a lot further gone than me in the sense of, like, people who had tried to kill themselves way too many times. And I was like, I'm going to surround myself either with no one, because I'm going to sleep at 10:00 P.M., or just more positive people, which I feel like is a really crummy thing to do, but I needed to do it."

Those who were in long-term romantic relationships often cited them as a factor contributing to an overall feeling of stability. "Part of what made me feel okay with stopping when I did was being in this sort of stable relationship," said Dana. Shannon said that her fiancé was a big help in her effort to get off antidepressants.

He's been exceptionally patient, and very understanding, and he's helped me work through it. He slowly helped push me out of my comfort zone, especially from an anxiety sense. He'll help to put me in a situation that would normally trigger my anxiety, usually social stuff, but he'll be there, and kind of assure me that everything's going to be okay.

—*Shannon, age twenty-six*

She also talked about the importance of social contact in general.

> I'm the first person to say that if you're depressed, or if you're anxious, the last thing you want to do is anything. You don't want to eat, you don't want to shower. You definitely don't want to go out on a hike or go to the mall or something like that. But you have to do something. Once you isolate yourself, that's when you've crossed over to letting it get you. Even if all you do is go for a walk, and say hi to one person that you pass during the walk, that's an accomplishment.
>
> —*Shannon, age twenty-six*

Several people described feeling as though they had become better at noticing their own needs and taking action to meet them—a combination of being both more vigilant and more relaxed. "I've worked out enough strategies so that I never get to the bottom anymore," said Isabel.

> I used to get into the thing where like, what I want to do is just, like, watch a movie, but that's bad because I should be trying to be productive, so I would spend the whole day not doing anything, and then end up feeling like I was a waste of a person. But now, I allow myself some, like, "Oh, if you want to chill out, that's cool, you can just chill out for an hour," and limit the number of things that I expect myself to do in a day. Which I often exceed. It's not that I have to struggle through all my days, but lowering my demands on myself has been big.   —*Isabel, age twenty-seven*

Isabel's comment is in line with the many ways people told me that the passage of time had often acted as a powerful intervention of its own. They talked about seeming to acquire a new resilience as they got older—as if living were a skill that they were improving at with age. Dana said she'd gained perspective. "Over the years, with medications and without, I've gotten so much better at not mistaking a negative mood for reality," she wrote in an e-mail. Alexa claimed she'd gotten better at putting herself first. Describing her sleep routine, she said, "The older I get, the more I'm like, 'I don't care if I'm boring, I just want to be healthy.'" These observations made perfect sense to me. By my midtwenties, I'd felt the same things: life did feel like it was getting a little easier as the years went by. All the emotions were still there, but even the strong ones weren't quite as jagged as they used to be.

The sense that life becomes easier to manage as we age hasn't gone entirely unnoticed by science. I felt tickled when I discovered a study in which psychological researchers who tracked hundreds of university graduates for seven years found that, on average, their subjects enjoyed a robust and significant decrease in depressive symptoms over the decade of their twenties.[5] Middle-aged people had even fewer depressive symptoms than twentysomethings, and they expressed less anger as well.[6] A psychologist who wasn't involved in the study hastened to tell me that the results shouldn't be taken as evidence that we "outgrow" depression, or that you can't get depressed at any age— and they aren't. But the study does lend credence to the idea that, old chestnuts about "the best years of your life" notwithstanding, most people begin to feel more calm and stable as they leave adolescence well behind.

Meghan, for one, told me she believes that being older has made life easier to deal with. "Definitely!" she said. "For sure."

My sister's in college right now, and she's a sophomore, and her experience is so similar to mine, and the fact that her capacity to handle stress is so little, or small, and she is having a really hard time, and she freaks out really hard sometimes in this sort of nihilistic way, like "I don't understand, and there is no point, I can't do anything," and it's really hard to hear her go through this, but I'm, part of me doesn't worry too much because just by getting older, I was better able to handle these things. So I imagine that she will be able to as well. But it's really hard! It just breaks your heart.

—*Meghan, age twenty-five*

WHEN I BEGAN tapering down on Zoloft in 2006, part of my bargain with myself was that I would abandon the project if I felt that it was necessary—that I was going to try to stay mindful of the difference between normal emotional ups and downs and the extra, grinding sensation of depression, and not force myself to suffer the latter just for the sake of being pill-free. During a spate of gray days in March, about six months after I'd gone off antidepressants completely, I started to wonder whether that time had come. I'd hit a low point at my job. A relationship had ended. We'd lost our lease on the apartment with the lovely cocoa-brown room and had moved to a neighborhood that seemed tougher, colder, farther flung. New York had done that thing that New York can do, whipping around on you, turning from bright and exciting to cruel and strident, like a trap you could get stuck in forever, or a playground bully who won't let you into the game.

Later that month, I went so far one week as to find a psychiatrist who accepted my new health plan, and steal away to her doily-strewn office on a lunch break. Over the course of a month or more, she tried me on a few things, including, at last, a tricyclic antidepressant that overstimulated me so much that she suggested I buy a bag of clear, empty pill capsules from a health food store, break apart the antidepressant capsules, and sweep a few grains of the powder into the clear caps, as a way of taking an infinitesimal dose. I did as she instructed. It may have helped, I don't remember. I do remember catching sight of myself a week or so later in the reflection of my darkened bedroom window, hunched over and working away like a pharmacist. I had one of those crystallizing moments. It suddenly felt to me that whatever I was doing, I was doing it prophylactically. I wasn't at the bottom, I was afraid of getting there. I felt overstimulated, disappointed, and sometimes lonely, I realized, but I didn't feel *sick*. And while I'd stayed on antidepressants in the past for less, this time I decided to take a bet on myself.

Days piled up, the same for a while, then different. One morning I woke up and instead of feeling dread or self-annoyance, I felt the simple pleasure of being focused on outward things: the touch of clean sheets on my skin; the sight of my new curtains, black and white this time, billowing in the early light. More time passed, and the grounded feeling stayed. I took the psychiatrist's last prescription out of my wallet and put it deep in a drawer.

Life still wasn't perfect, but after that, it turned. Whatever it had been—the end of a romance, adjustment to a world past academia, the long New York City winter, or a little bit of each—the cycle came to an end, and one by one the areas of trouble worked their way toward resolution. I remembered what John had said in our therapy sessions the year before about the value of aggression, and I tried my best to take action, go after what I wanted, and change all the bothersome things I could.

In the winter of 2007, I reached the end of a year which, aside from that early-spring flirtation, I'd spent completely without medication. It was the first such year I'd had since I was eighteen. In my journal, I wrote that while it hadn't been an easy time, it had felt like an empowering one. Realizing that I could feel bad for a while and then recover satisfied me deeply in some way. It increased my confidence to know that the things I'd learned would make me feel better still had an effect, even without the net of antidepressants. Most of all, I felt glad to have finally answered to my own satisfaction that old mystery, the question of what I would be like without medication. If there was an irony, it lay in how non-cataclysmic the answer was. Month in and month out, as far as I can tell, the person I am off antidepressants isn't so very different from the person I am on them. It may be silly that I had to go to great lengths to accept in my bones what psychiatrists have been saying all along. But I did have to, and the knowledge in my bones feels invaluable.

The hope that getting off of antidepressants would somehow perfect me, that I'd zoom to new heights of creativity, or clarity of thought, or personal charm, were laid to rest. But that's all right. The fears that I'd completely fall apart were put down too. I wrote at the time that somehow, knowing that the difference antidepressants make is less profound than I had sometimes imagined would make me feel more peaceful about taking them again, if I ever decided to. They wouldn't challenge my sense of self the way they had when I was in my teens and early twenties.

As my year without antidepressants came to an end, I didn't

have any immediate plans to get back on them. Five years later, I still don't. Not taking medication has become routine, a habit that feels as ingrained as taking it used to be. That's not to say that I don't sometimes think about going back. I agree somewhat with Grace, who, when I asked her whether life was easier to manage now, said:

> Not really, no! [Laughs.] I mean, I think. Not really. It's still just as hard. I think I'm less dramatic about it, certainly. I allow myself less drama. But when I think back on it, I still have the same problems that I did, the same things still drive me crazy. —*Grace, age thirty-four*

I do feel like life has gotten easier to manage, but I relate to the sense that while time and experience dial them back, old issues never truly disappear. And sometimes—in February, or after a breakup, or during a period of stomach-knotting stress at work—I ask myself whether another way might be better. I consider the possibility that I'm pushing myself to prove a point, or wonder whether I've been living inside a low-grade depression for ages without even recognizing it. Once or twice, I've even been back to look at the DSM-IV criteria for depression. Each time, I've realized I'm nowhere close.

MOST OF THE people I talked to who used antidepressants are glad they did. "Lexapro was my stepping-stone," said Shannon. "It was the thing that kept me alive, that made me realize I'm capable of being a human being." Isabel said that "at the time, when I first went on medication in high school, I didn't know what to do. I didn't have any resources in myself to help myself feel better.

Medication was like a raft." Plenty said they'd be willing to go back on antidepressants if they felt they needed to. Some specifically defended others' choices to use them. "Even though I'm not on them, I'm [down on] anyone who accuses anyone on meds of being weak, or whatever," said Alexa, "because to me, that is just not understanding." Maybe surprisingly, most acknowledged that life without antidepressants is a little bit harder than life with them. But they find that they are able to bear the difference, and they often said that they gain a sense of meaning from their choice that makes the extra difficulty seem worthwhile.

Christine, thirty-six, who had stopped taking antidepressants six months earlier on the advice of her psychiatrist in Denmark, said that she valued the emotionality she has when she is not on medication. "He said, 'There's nothing wrong with you clinically, and I think we should just stop.'"

> So I stopped, and he was pretty right. Of course I can feel that the world has kind of stepped one step closer to me, where I start crying a little more often now—but it's nice, because my sensitivity has come back, and so far, it's been okay. —*Christine, age thirty-six*

Alexa said that while living without medication was tougher in some ways, she liked the feeling of being able to accommodate her natural tendencies, instead of trying to change them. When she stopped using antidepressants, she said, "I totally felt these problems come back, these problems that had not even developed in my teenage years. I'm definitely an anxious person. And when I came off, I was like this person who's always a little bit too up or a little bit too down, not proportionate to reality."

And I haven't come to peace with that in the sense that I
like it all the time, but there are ways to manage it besides
being on drugs for me. And I guess I try to see the upside
of it. Like, being a little up is kind of fun, because I become
more creative, I have energy to make things. And then being
a little down kind of sucks, but I feel like I'm the kind of
person who's always on the go, and when I get down I try to
think of it as like, My body needs to rest, or like, I need to
take it easy; I'm going to have a day where I read in bed.

—*Alexa, age twenty-three*

David, thirty-one, quit under duress; he tried for years to
make medication work, but all of the many medications he used
eventually caused him to become manic or created other side
effects that made it impossible to for him continue. He told me
that, on balance, he's sorry that medication hasn't worked for
him. But he also takes pride in the way he has learned to manage
without. When we talked, he had been off of everything for over
a year. "And I'm doing okay," he said. In an e-mail, he elaborated:

I'm not the whirlwind of productive energy I wish I was, but
I do okay at my job, I have a fairly busy social life, I carry
through moderately ambitious projects outside of work, I'm
moving forward in my career. And I've come to accept that
the person I wish I was is not someone I can be, at least not
for longer than a couple days, a week at most. But for me,
it has always been borrowing against something, in terms
of both emotions and energy level. So let it level out: I'm
always going to be introverted, and slightly nervous, and
self-critical, and slightly scattered, and easily distracted.

But I can almost like that, or at least appreciate it as a viable alternative to the people I have been in the past.

—*David, age thirty-one*

This type of thinking won't make sense to everyone. Isabel told me that her mother, like most of her other family members, has been on antidepressants for years. "My mother and I are very close," said Isabel. "And she couldn't understand why I would ever want to stop taking medication. Her philosophy about everything is, 'Why be in pain? Why not just play it safe? The thing makes you feel better, so why not just do what makes you feel better?' And medication has been such a blessing for her life, that she can't understand why people wouldn't want to take it. So, for a long time—and only recently did she stop doing this—when I was upset, she would be like, 'Well, maybe you should just try to go back on the drugs for a while.'"

Other people who are drawn to the idea of quitting will discover that it isn't practical for them. While I think that self-care and lifestyle changes can make a big difference, I know they're not a panacea. As a personal reminder, I sometimes think back to a moment that occurred near the end of my time in California. I was at the Berkeley YMCA, trying to "manage" my need for medication with exercise, in the last week or two before I packed it in and called the psychiatrist. A few weeks later, when I was feeling better, I tried to wring a little humor out of the memory by saying to myself, *Okay, when you're doing exercise to try to feel better, and you're actually crying* while *you're doing the exercise* (crunches for me, if I remember), *maybe that's a signal that it's time to bring out the big guns.* I have a friend who had a therapist who once told her that depression is when you feel like it's almost impossibly effortful to get through the things you need to do. By the same token, keeping yourself in an acceptable frame of mind shouldn't feel like an exhausting, full-time job, let alone one you're slowly failing at.

Maybe this starts to get us back to a sense of why quitting medication has been and still is a delicate topic. The issue can confront us with an unfairness: it's something that is possible for some people but not possible, and certainly not advisable, for all. It's delicate because it is tempting to read one person's choice to forego medication as an editorial comment on the validity of the decisions of others. It is also touchy because it confronts us with the vision of people making themselves suffer to secure an outcome that they want—the possibility that the choice to quit will be guided more by a stigma against medication than a clear-eyed assessment of what is right in a given situation. Finally, it's delicate because it requires making judgment calls about what is and isn't normal to feel, calls that may be easy at the far ends of the spectrum but, toward the middle, are difficult enough to make for oneself and very uncomfortable to try to apply to other people. No wonder the question of stopping has been one that we've often preferred not to talk about. But we need to find a way to, and we may find that the subject becomes less forbidding the more we try.

As Meghan discovered, sometimes it is possible to change the story that you are telling about yourself. But at other times, just wanting to tell a different story about oneself does not make it feasible, or even a good idea. Quitting becomes problematic when your desire to fit your life into a certain narrative starts to cloud your ability to see things as they are. The few times during these interviews when I became uncomfortable were the times when I began to get the feeling that someone was trying too hard—that their quitting seemed to have more to do with a wish to bring their life in line with an identity that they wanted to take on than it did with attention to how things were actually going for them.

Conversely, the quitting stories I felt best about were the ones in which someone described a choice that felt, in the truest sense, free—as if it were made in the absence of a need to secure one outcome or the other. I felt comfortable when I was talking to people who seemed able to balance their gladness about not being on medication anymore with a sense that this gladness wasn't essential to them—it was something extra and nice, but not central to their ability to value themselves as a person. It is a delicate balance to achieve, one I thought that Dana put very well. When I asked her in a follow-up e-mail how she thought that growing up on antidepressants had affected her, and whether she would make the same treatment choices over again, she replied:

> It's quite possible that without medication, I would have been too depressed and anxious and unsure of myself to go to college 2,500 miles from home or spend a semester in Australia or have love affairs with cool and strange men or move to New York after graduation or make it through the first two years of graduate school. I might have used more drugs and alcohol instead of less. I might have become more socially withdrawn. I might have thought even more about killing myself. I can't know, but it feels very possible.
>
> So, no, I wouldn't change a thing. The choice was mine from the start. I exercised my independence (perhaps unwisely) over and over again by going on and off the meds

as I saw fit. The past three years have demonstrated to me that I can live life and weather enormous stress without the medication—I emerged neither physically nor psychologically dependent. In my estimation, the medication served me well and did me no harm. And I'm happy where I am.

—*Dana, age thirty-one*

9 | CONVERTS

s I moved into the second half of my twenties, taking a considered break from antidepressants seemed like a reasonable thing to try; when it turned out to be supportable, I decided it was something that I wanted to continue. In the last chapter, I described a handful of people who performed a similar maneuver. As they left college days and quarter-life crises behind them, they felt pulled to experiment with leaving medication behind too, and the move often felt valuable and right to them. But as I continued with my interviews, I also noticed a countervailing pattern. Some people, even those who felt diffident about antidepressants when they were younger, find that they become more committed to using medication as time goes on. People who stick with antidepressants or return to them a little later in life often find new ways to think and talk about medication that allow them to feel a greater sense of control than they did at first. They replace the worries that many younger people have, about how antidepressants might alienate them from their real selves, with a sense that antidepressants are a tool they can use deliberately to achieve a way of life that is right for them.

At first, James seemed an unlikely candidate for a champion

of antidepressants. His stories about medication had much more to do with the things that medications hadn't done for him than the things they had. The failure wasn't for lack of effort. "I'm what's considered 'treatment-resistant,'" he said. "Very, very, very treatment-resistant." Early in our interview, James explained to me patiently that he'd been on medication for most of the last half of his thirty-two years. All in all, he had tried forty-seven different drugs, singly and in a mind-boggling array of combinations. "With that amount of effort," he said with a small sigh, "most people would have found something that worked."

James was tall and broad-shouldered, with a neatly trimmed brown beard and the precise amount of extra poundage that, on a man, invites teddy bear comparisons. He was a web developer by trade, and put his words together with a degree of precision that gave his speech a slightly formal air. James said he had been aware of depression as a force in his life for almost as long as he could remember. School officials first commented on his "issues of sadness and anger" when he was six. At fifteen, he carried out what he described as a "major suicide attempt," swallowing a massive overdose of his family members' prescription drugs. He was found unconscious and rushed to the hospital where, he noted matter-of-factly, "I actually literally did die for four minutes." Afterward, James spent several months in the hospital—in the waning days of the 1980s, long hospital stays underwritten by insurance were still common.

Though he'd been depressed for a long time, the hospital stay was James's first entrance into the mental health care system. James's attending physician in the hospial put him on Prozac, then still a new and exciting drug. As James recalled, Prozac made him anxious at first, but over a few weeks its effects faded away to nothing. But he vividly remembered feeling hostile toward the idea of taking Prozac. "I was afraid of the stigma, and what it said about me. Even though I'd been hospitalized for so long, the idea of taking meds seemed to solidify the idea that I was crazy," he said. "What's going on in my head isn't visible, but me taking a pill is much more tangible to the world." When he was transferred upon his release to a new psychiatrist who took him off of Prozac, he felt immensely relieved.

James didn't try medication again until he was nineteen, when a second suicide attempt forced him to withdraw from college. "It was nowhere near as bad [as the first one]," he said. "Technically it was a very good-looking cry for help." Still, it was alarming to James, and to his parents too. James moved home, got a job, and began working intensively with a psychiatrist to find a medication or a combination of medications that would help. For six years, he tried one drug after another, with a lack of success that reached almost epic proportions. James had side effects major, minor, and nearly unheard of. On the mood stabilizer Depakote, he said, he packed on extra weight that he hasn't been able to shed since. "Either I had a side effect from a drug, or it didn't work, that was the pattern," said James. "It was a merry-go-round of absolutely nothing."

Part of the reason he is such a challenging case, James explained, is that he suffers from major depression on top of atypical depression—a more chronic condition, which is marked by symptoms that include oversleeping (James's record is thirty-one hours straight, though ten to twelve hours a night is normal for him), overeating, and a sensation of heaviness approaching paralysis in the limbs. It is also characterized by rejection sensitivity so extreme that the atypical depressive often avoids forming close social bonds. James told me that although he's dated women in the past, it is "an unusual thing for me," and while he is comfortable enough in group social settings, and enjoys them, he has a hard time making friends. "I have one friend," he said. "He's an excellent friend. He's been my friend for six years. I was the best man at his wedding." For the most part, though, James said, "I'm so afraid of rejection that I don't make connections." Over the years, medication would occasionally chip away at the symptoms of James's major depression, but it always left his atypical symptoms untouched.

James's low opinion of antidepressants remained unchanged until, in the aftermath of a third suicide attempt at twenty-five, he began seeing a new psychiatrist who quickly hit upon a cocktail of drugs that affected James in ways that he had scarcely believed possible. "I felt *great*," said James. "Just truly great. I can almost give you the exact dates. I mean, I was still neurotic; the stuff that had happened to me in my childhood was still there, but the physiological aspect of the depression was totally gone. I felt a way I hadn't felt since I was three. It was miraculous." His atypical symptoms were banished too; in fact, James first noticed the drugs were working during the holiday party of a company he contracted for. "I suddenly realized I wasn't nervous," he said. "There were no barriers. I even flirted with a girl."

Four months later, James was hanging out at a bar with his cousin when he realized he didn't feel well. That night, he developed a high fever and checked himself into the emergency room. "When I came out, [the medications] weren't working anymore," he said. "They had just stopped. What had been there for four months was gone." And though he has continued to search even more aggressively for effective medications since then, he has never had a comparable drug effect again.

By now, said James, he has tried every SSRI, every SNRI, and most of the antipsychotics and mood stabilizers. He has used a medication that is not for sale in the United States, which his pharmacologist, who is regarded as one of the best in James's city, brought back from Europe in his luggage. He pins hope on a handful of medications he hasn't tried yet, medications I had never heard of; next, he said, he wants to sample an MAOI that is available in a transdermal formulation, like the nicotine patches people use to quit smoking. In the meantime, he attends therapy and copes as best he can. For years he worked part time and went to college at night. He finally finished his undergraduate degree and hopes to attend a professional program someday. When we met, though, James had been receiving disability for several years. He was cycling out of a major depressive episode and hadn't worked in a while, though he'd recently heard about a part-time opportunity through a family member, which he hoped to follow up on soon.

Given the ratio of success to failure in James's medication story, you might expect him to be furious with pharmaceuticals, but he isn't. In fact he's a vocal believer in the importance of medication (given his failures, he said, "I think drugs are even more important for other people than they are for me."), and he's unflinchingly dedicated to continuing to search for medication that will work for him again. In large part, the four months of success when he was twenty-five were the fulcrum around which James's opinion of medication turned, the conversion experience that solidified his faith in the drug approach. "In some ways, those four months are very good and they're very bad," he said. "They show me what I'm missing, but they also remind me what's possible. I can't imagine having gotten to forty-seven meds without knowing that it's possible that they could work."

But he also attributed his evolved attitude to changes in himself. Part of it was getting older. When he first started Prozac at fifteen, James was preoccupied with what his classmates would think of him. "What you think as a teenager is very different from what you think as an adult," he said. "I already had fears about being weird or being a nerd; anything extra was scary, and something that I couldn't allow myself to do or really accept." For another thing, James came to take his problems more seriously over time. "After the second suicide attempt at eighteen, the idea that I might continue to have suicide attempts was scary," James said. "When I'm not suicidal, I don't want to die." Still, it was years more before he became invested in medication as something he actively felt like he wanted to do, on his own behalf and no one else's. "Once upon a time, my parents' approval was ridiculously important to me," he remembered. "There was a period of time where part of the reason I was okay with meds was because my parents wanted me to take meds, because they were scared of what I could do to myself without them. So that was part of the change." He went on:

Eventually, the change became all my own, and their opinion stopped mattering. Part of it was those four months, when I was given a taste of what life can be like. Prior to that, I was trying out of fear and out of desire to please my parents. It wasn't until I was twenty-five that I truly became convinced that at least I need to try. There's no harm in trying. You get a side effect, it's a bitch, you get off the drug and it goes away. It's not the end of the world. And I'll take the gamble of getting an annoying side effect that I get rid of just by going off the drug, for the potential of one day finding the combination that no longer puts roadblocks in the work I need to do in therapy.

One thing that sank in as I listened to James tell his story was the extent to which the questions that have coalesced around antidepressants for me, and for some of the people whose antidepressant stories I relate to the most, were almost completely irrelevant in his case. For years I'd concerned myself with the relationship of antidepressants to identity, the ambiguity of the border between normal moods and disordered ones, and the issue of need in cases where need might legitimately be considered ambiguous. These weren't bad questions to ask—they were the ones that experience had brought me, and I knew from my conversations that many had shared them—but in talking to James I realized afresh that they are, in a very real sense, luxury questions. Worrying about the finer points of antidepressant use, like what it means to your sense of self, is a privilege denied to those for whom the pills never fulfill their basic promise in the first place. And they are not likely to be top concerns for people who are dealing with a whole other order of problem. There is nothing like talking to someone who finds it hard to hold down a job or flirt with a girl—someone who, when he says he has trouble getting out of bed in the morning, means something very different from what you have meant, the times when you've complained about having trouble getting out of bed in the morning—to make you feel churlish for how much time you've spent wondering whether antidepressants have tempered your personality. In James's presence I started to feel a little like a woman at a fancy restaurant, sending back the soup because there was a fly in it, while people like James were pressing their noses against the window, daydreaming about a square meal. There wasn't much I could do about the situation except stop to take note of the perspective it offered. James's experience had made him viscerally sure of the thing it had been my good fortune to be able to dither about; at this point in his life, he felt certain that anything he might have to lose by using medication pales in comparison to what he has to gain.

MANY PEOPLE WHO came to feel more positive about antidepressants over time talked, in one way or another, about a sense of agency. They began to focus less on their fears about what uncontrollable things medication might be doing to them, and more on the active, empowering dimensions of their choice to use medication in the first place. Denise, twenty-seven, used antidepressants in college and after, for about five years in all, but she said it was a habit she'd always felt ambivalent about. Her family didn't really approve of medication ("My father is manic-depressive," she said, "but he won't take meds because they 'make his tummy hurt.'"), and Denise wasn't too sure what she thought about them either.

"I think that a lot of my depression comes out of anxiety, and isolation too," she said, explaining that she had been living independently for a long time; she moved out on her own when she was sixteen and put herself through community college, before transferring to a four-year school. She lived off campus, and her college boyfriend became her connection to the rest of her social life at school. After college and before her move to New York City, Denise recalled becoming "very upset and clingy with friends." Her doctor gave her a prescription for the antidepressant Lexapro. "It was just my G.P.," she said, adding that she had wanted him to prescribe Xanax, for anxiety, but that he had seemed unwilling to do so (Xanax is technically a controlled substance). In the end, Denise ended up taking Lexapro for four years, but she never felt that it had a pronounced effect. She knew it was an antidepressant, and she had never considered depression to be her main problem. "I just don't feel that Lexapro did anything for me, in terms of anxiety," she told me. Eventually, she took herself off it.

When I met her, Denise had started using antidepressants again just the month before—but this time, she said, her outlook on them was completely different. Earlier that year, she'd gone through a breakup, a familiar trigger for her "separation anxiety and abandonment issues." "When I'm living on my own, or starting a new job, I'm very self-sufficient, so even though it's hard, I'll muddle through," she said. "But when a relationship doesn't work, something kicks into gear." She began to feel anxious, lonely, and sad, and she also started losing weight, which frightened her because she has a history of anorexia and is afraid, every time she begins to shed weight, that she'll get carried away by the temptation to lose even more.

Getting depressed and anxious on the heels of a breakup wasn't new to Denise, but she told me that she'd deliberately decided to respond in a new way this time. She said that she was using the end of the relationship as an opportunity to take a good hard look at her life, and make changes. When she was honest, she continued, she had to admit that even though her depressions were often brought on by life events, there was something about life that had felt off in between the crises too. "The best thing about the end of this past relationship is that it's making me realize how low I've been, because that's what I've been attracting into my life," she said. "As far as the hard part about the end of this relationship, I feel like there's this huge void, and that void had always been there; it's just that by burying it in work or in a relationship you sort of forget about it. So it's made me realize that I've always felt pretty low, and that there's something I need to do to up myself and attract more positive things into my life." She even told me that she thought taking Lexapro had been abetting her apathy in a way—that it had helped her limp along without addressing the things that were really bothering her. "I think part of the reason I was taking it was that part of me knew I was depressed, but I still wasn't doing anything about it in terms of therapy or anything like that."

Denise said that returning to antidepressants was part of a bigger decision to start taking her mental well-being seriously. She began by finding a therapist who helped her locate a new doctor, a specialist with more medication expertise than her old G.P. "This is the first time I've seen a psychiatrist where I feel like he's going to get me on the right meds, and I'm going to report back to him, and if I don't feel any improvement, he's going to change things," Denise said. "He was very concerned about how we got along together, which was great. He wanted to make sure that we had a good rapport, so he could feel like I was opening up to him, and giving him all the right details so that he could recommend the right kind of drugs."

But Denise also said she was no longer content with a medication-only approach. In fact, she was setting out on an almost gleefully eclectic program to revamp her life, sampling a multitude of techniques for feeling better and intending to hang on to the ones that worked. Medication, therapy, an alternative anxiety-reduction technique called E.F.T., Buddhist meditation classes, a support group for people with mood disorders, a psychic, a new online-dating profile, scheduled social activities with friends—Denise was trying a little bit of everything. While not everyone will agree with the effectiveness of all these approaches, to Denise the important thing was her new sense of resolve. Earlier, she said, she'd been floating along, taking Lexapro "out of habit" and not really facing the problems she knew were there. This time, taking medication felt to her like an active choice, part of a larger personal commitment to taking care of herself as well as she can. When I asked Denise whether she'd ever had negative feelings about antidepressants, her answer illuminated the shift in her thinking. "Yeah, definitely," she said.

That's one of the reasons I got off antidepressants this past summer. Because I was feeling like, "Oh yeah, I'm fine." And there's a stigma attached to it. I'm from a Scandinavian background, and Scandinavians are very stoic, they tend not to talk about a lot of things. Now I'm feeling like, with my background and my family history, and the way I'm reacting to certain life events, I definitely need to be on them. But it's more just realizing they're a tool, not a solution. So I just sort of get my mood up, and I keep experimenting with life and figuring out what makes me happy and how to handle it better. Part of it is me shifting my life philosophy around, but I'm hoping that the meds keep it that way, no matter what happens.

At twenty-seven, Denise said, she felt like she needed to start taking the same kind of responsibility for her emotional life that she had long been used to doing in the world of school and work. "I feel like I'm on my own," she said. "I don't have a family. I have close friends, but they're scattered all over the place, so I feel like I'm on my own, which creates a lot of anxiety and issues. But I also feel like I'm teaching myself a lot of things. I'm introspective. I know what's wrong. And I feel like I can do something about it."

FOR DENISE, A big part of feeling better about using medication was finding a doctor she could communicate with. In fact, improved relationships with doctors were a theme running through the stories of people who stayed on antidepressants. An alarming number of the people I talked to described having adversarial feelings about psychiatrists, particularly in their younger days. "I've never had a good interaction with a psychiatrist," said Alexa, twenty-four. "Not meaning they were mean to me, but they don't look at you as human." Sophia, twenty, said she didn't like entrusting herself to "psychiatrists who don't know who I am, anyway. My last psychiatrist forgot I was anorexic! He asked me how the OCD was." Nathan, thirty-one, remembered feeling objectified by psychiatrists' diagnostic labels. "Once you're put into that hole, that category, I don't feel like curing the person is even something that enters the doctor's head anymore."

Others, though, reported that their relationships with doctors improved over time; as they got older, they learned what they liked and didn't like in a doctor-patient relationship, and came to feel that they had more power in the exchange. Heather, thirty-nine, said that she had a string of psychiatrists in her teens and twenties whom she disliked or found ineffective—but that by now, she'd become much better at picking doctors who will give her the care she needs. "Now I feel like I'm pretty much an expert at it," she said. "I can tell immediately if I like a doctor or not. I had a doctor not that long ago who had a fancy office with Oriental rugs. He had a scale, every time you went he would weigh you, he'd type everything into his computer. But I was on something, some medicine, and I was on too much of it; my hands were trembling all up my whole arm, and I was just like, 'I feel crazy with this arm shake.' I'd complain about it a bunch of times and he was just like, 'No no, stay on it, we're doing good.' A lot of doctors don't want to mess up their track record by listening to the patient [and changing] the medication again. And then I stopped going to him, and got another doctor I'm going to now, and he is good. If that much is off, he's going to change it up for you."

Denise also wasn't the only person who described medications as a "tool." The word popped up again and again, particularly among people who'd once felt dubious about using them. For these people, the word *tool* was a metaphor that allowed them to feel a greater sense of agency around medication: to think of an antidepressant as a tool is a way to emphasize the power that the user of the drug has over the decision to take it, and de-emphasize the idea that the drug might be controlling its user instead. "I didn't like the idea of having my mood, my feelings, in some way my personality—I mean, that's how I thought at the time—depend on some kind of drug," said Elizabeth, twenty-five, about when she started to take antidepressants at fifteen, "because it felt creepy, and scary, and yeah, artificial." She often felt "like I'm admitting defeat if I'm taking medication, like I can't deal with something myself." But, she continued, "I do see it differently now. I think there's something to be said for the idea that if you can help take the load off, if there's some kind of medication that works and helps you feel better, it is so much easier to climb out of a hole if you already have a shovel."

Mia, an outspoken twenty-three year old, highlighted the role of language and metaphor in her own tempestuous relationship with medication. Mia described herself as a strong critic of "the mainstream mental-health system," which she blamed for making her feel "broken and bad and wrong and Other and all these things" when her mother first started taking her to psychiatrists at age thirteen. After ten years of involvement with that system, Mia spoke of it in somewhat jaded terms. While she didn't deny that her mother had reason to be concerned, she said that she was often nonplussed by the care she'd gotten. "I have been on every medication under the sun," she said. "I've been diagnosed with everything from depression to anxiety to bipolar. I had a severe eating disorder in high school. I was diagnosed as borderline by one guy, I mean just endless anything—PTSD, body dysmorphic disorder, all these different disorders. And 'Let's blast things on her and give her drugs' was sort of the thinking. Just a slew of chemical cocktails, from age thirteen till now."

But despite being critical of the mental health system, Mia had to admit that she'd also benefited from that system. Like a lot of people she knows, she said, she struggles to balance the fact that "I hate the idea that something chemical could be helping me" with feeling that medication is useful or even necessary for her. While she cited a lot of sources of solace in her life, such as "learning how to eat well, and building community, and getting involved in activism and organizing when I got to college, especially around mental health and women's mental health," she also allowed that "I think the different medications I've been on, antianxiety, antidepressants, antipsychotics, some have saved my life at moments; I'm not going to say they didn't."

Mia said that over time, largely thanks to her activism and her reading, she'd become interested in how language and narrative shape experience. Gradually, she had devised a way of talking and thinking about herself that allowed her to take what she wanted from psychiatry and leave the rest behind. She said that she chooses to think of her problems as being tightly enmeshed with her personality. "I am an incredibly emotionally intense person," she said. "I feel things deeply and strongly." While she was comfortable seeking treatment, she refused to accept a narrative about being "ill" or "sick," preferring to think of medication as something that she uses to manage her sometimes difficult temperament rather than something she uses to treat a disease. (She told me that while she identifies with many aspects of the DSM-IV description of the mental disorder known as bipolar II, she is careful to make a fine distinction: "I am *not* bipolar II. I *have* bipolar II *tendencies*.")

Mia's philosophy has led her to invent her own style of interacting with mental health practitioners. "Whenever I go to start a new relationship with a new provider of whatever sort," she said, "they're a provider to me, they're not—perhaps they are a doctor, but they're not treating me, they're not *fixing* me, they're not fixing a problem."

I don't like to think of my experiences as problems, as illnesses. I have experiences; I'm sensitive, I'm intense, I'm passionate, I'm fiery. I am not broken. I say "crazy" with a very loving spin on it. I don't like being identified as a patient. And so when I'm interacting with someone and they call me a patient, I tell them, "I'm a client here. I am a consumer, and I'm consuming your services." I am coming to you, and what these words mean to me is that I want to interact with you as someone who is giving me a service. Just like I am not the patient of an acupuncturist, I am not the patient of the psychiatrist. You have a resource that I find helpful, so I am asking you for it. But that doesn't mean that I am in your power. It's not about "I am weak, and I am needy." At times I feel weak and needy. But what I choose to do with that is an empowered choice, even in my weakness.

—*Mia, age twenty-three*

OF ALL THE antidepressant stories that I heard, Anastasia's provided the fullest example of the many adjustments that can lead a person from feeling that medication is hampering the self to feeling that it is supporting it. Anastasia was thirty-five, with big blue eyes, and curly brown hair stuffed loosely under a sporty stocking cap. She grew up in San Francisco, the only child of two college professors who separated when she was young. In person, she made a number of impressions at once, striking me as a unique blend of sharp, restless, idealistic, sensitive, tender, angry.

Like James and Denise, Anastasia reported that her early experiences with medication were mixed. She first began taking antidepressants in the midst of a rough transition out of college. "At college I had felt smart, I had felt validated, I had felt important," she said—but figuring out how to enter the larger world with that sense of self intact was anything but obvious. After graduation, she continued, "I moved to Seattle, where I didn't know a soul, and I was trying to figure out how to be myself in the world and I didn't really know how to do that, in the working world." Anastasia had studied fine art in school and eventually found a job working at a large commercial photography studio. The position was administrative, and the work didn't provide Anastasia with any of the good feelings she remembered and missed from school.

Anastasia had been feeling low even before she took the job, and as the months went by, she became more and more severely depressed. "I was having to do this whole thing of going to work and pretending that I was okay, which was becoming almost intolerable," she said. Her relationships with her coworkers, never good to begin with, worsened as she had a harder time concealing how upset she was and how much she resented her job. Laughing a little at the memory, Anastasia explained that when she found herself sometimes wearing a certain knit hat to the office, because she liked to imagine that it afforded her some kind of psychic protection from the toxic work environment, she decided it was time to take some action.

At the time, Anastasia had a therapist who recommended that she try an antidepressant; he referred her to a psychiatrist who got her started on Zoloft. "[Zoloft] allowed me to function at my job," Anastasia recalled. "But it definitely didn't lift me to any very tolerable level. It just sort of made it easier for me not to want to kill everybody at work and storm out in the middle of the day." In fact Anastasia often resented Zoloft because she felt that it might be making her able to put up with a situation that she would have preferred not to be in at all. "I remember feeling a certain kind of anger," she said, "and worrying, like, I used to joke that I was taking the drugs so I could keep the job. And there was something that seemed very wrong about that to me, for obvious reasons. You know, 'Why should I be working at a job that I have to take an antidepressant to tolerate?'" In a way, she felt like Emily, the writer who believed that Prozac made it possible for her to perform in her career, but with one crucial difference—Anastasia believed that Zoloft was supporting a life that she wanted no part of.

Eventually Anastasia quit, took another job that she didn't find so oppressive, and stopped using Zoloft. A couple of years had passed but, she said, she still hadn't put down roots in Seattle the way she had hoped to. ("There were a lot of people that I would go to a bar with or a show with," she recalled, "but I didn't have that many intimate friendships.") Her transition out of college still felt incomplete, and her career direction uncertain. She decided to spend some time traveling around the country, with the idea that a trip might give her time to do some thinking about herself and the future; she said she conceived of it as a "delayed adolescence."

Things began to go wrong before she even left town. During the planning stages, "I fell into a state of being paralyzed and unable to make a decision about where I was going to go, so I started temping," Anastasia remembered. "At this point, I wasn't seeing a psychiatrist and I wasn't taking meds, and I fell into an even deeper hole, where I was temping part-time and the rest of the time I was in my apartment, which was all packed up to leave, but I couldn't leave; I was in suspended animation. Eventually I got out and went traveling around the country. I was riding around on buses and sleeping on people's couches, except I was so distressed that I began to sort of think of myself as homeless. I was acting free and easy, but I was actually feeling really tormented." The more she traveled, the more lost, illegitimate, and indecisive she felt. After several months all over the U.S. and Central America, "I ended up on a friend's couch back in Seattle. I hit a wall and I was like, 'I don't know what to do with myself. I don't know how to stop moving around. I don't know where to live.' I felt like I had lost my whole internal compass somehow."

Like James and Denise, Anastasia was having an experience that would make her reassess her need for help. Using money that she had inherited when her grandfather died, Anastasia decided to check herself into a residential treatment program in the Northwest that she'd heard about during her time in Seattle. She stayed at the program for two months, and called her choice to go there "one of the best decisions I have ever made in my life." At the treatment center, she worked with a psychiatrist who put her back on Zoloft and also on an atypical antipsychotic called Zyprexa, which Anastasia remembers as "kind of a miracle drug for me at the time. It got me out of the state of total paralyzed hysteria I'd been in for months." Just as important, Anastasia said, the act of deciding to go into treatment made a difference in itself. "It got me moving," she said, "and it created this internal sense of 'I am taking this seriously, and I am doing something about it; my health is important to me.' So I think the statement that I made to myself by doing that is part of what was healing about it."

Going into treatment changed Anastasia's attitude about medication, which she went from seeing as something she was using to make a bad situation tolerable, to something that she could do to create a better situation on her own behalf and no one else's. She has continued to use medication since. Her experience hasn't been trouble-free. She has reshuffled her regimen many times, often to try to minimize side effects; drugs in Zyprexa's family are especially known to cause weight gain and metabolic changes. ("I used to make a joke, when I was on an antidepressant and a mood stabilizer," Anastasia said, "that the mood stabilizer made me chubby, but luckily it didn't matter because the Zoloft killed my sex drive, so you know, if I wasn't appealing to anyone, I wouldn't have to worry about wanting to be.")

Like Mia, Anastasia has also wondered how to square the fact that she benefits from medication with the fact that she often feels critical of mainstream psychiatry, and especially doesn't like diagnostic labels. For one thing, her symptoms, while sometimes severe, never fit neatly into a DSM category. For another thing, she has read widely in sociology and is inclined to be skeptical about the validity of such divisions. "Part of me struggles a little bit with the whole categorization process," she said, talking about support group meetings in which she's felt pressured to identify with a particular label, like unipolar or bipolar, and articulate an understanding of herself as a person who has a disease. "I have really mixed feelings about the utility of those kinds of labels for people, and their process of surviving," she said. "I think that sometimes a notion of being ill can be helpful, but I also think it can be harmful." When I asked her to frame her understanding of her own problems, she told me that she thinks they are related to an inborn excess of sensitivity, a "capacity for feeling deeply and for feeling pain" that can be problematic, but also beneficial in the right context. "I've always avoided practitioners who are really interested in understanding things in terms of illness and labels," she said. "I've shied away from that model."

Even so, Anastasia has found a way to feel comfortable with her own use of medication, and she gently but firmly disagrees with those who suggest that she doesn't need it. When we talked, she'd been seeing a psychiatrist who had recently wanted to get her off everything; she described him as "a Buddhist" and said "whatever, it's nice that he thinks that," but she insisted that now is not a good time for her to try stopping. She described her attitude toward medication as utilitarian; like Denise and Elizabeth, she understands medication as a tool she wields to get the results she needs. "Sometimes people I know, who are not on medication themselves, but have depression issues," she said,

will talk to me and get on their high horse about not being on medication, or how I don't need to be, or will talk to me about how I'm getting fucked by the pharmaceutical industry, and I take that argument only so far. I mean, I think that pharmaceutical companies are very interested in fucking people; I don't believe that they're these benevolent forces. On the other hand, I'm looking out for myself and I'm looking out for how to function, and if my goal is to function, then I'm going to use what I can from them to the best of my ability. So I just view it in terms of utility, whether it's working for me. And for me I just feel that unless I were in treatment all the time, or in a cozy, you know, *farmhouse*—I often feel like the world is too much for me, and this provides me some kind of protection.

Over time, Anastasia has come to see medication as a balancing act. A good medication regimen is one that allows her to feel like herself while also affording her the degree of protection that she feels like she needs. To illustrate the point, she told me about her recent time on Abilify, another atypical antipsychotic that a psychiatrist recently tried adding to her treatment. "Abilify was *amazing* in terms of my mood," she said. "Like, unbelievable. I was so nondepressed. I've never *been* so nondepressed. Normally, there's always part of me that's dragging my heels, and just wants to curl up in bed; the world often feels, at least on a small level, exhausting to me. But when I was taking Abilify I was like, 'I'm gonna take three subways to go work out! I'm gonna go dig a ditch fifty feet long and fifty feet deep!'" There were only two problems. One was physical; she could hardly sleep. But the other was more personal and aesthetic. Anastasia felt like she couldn't relate to the person she was on Abilify. She confided to her therapist that when she was on Abilify, she "almost didn't remember what it felt like to feel bad. I really could not even *imagine* what depression felt like anymore. Which sounds like, 'Well, that's weird, why would you care?' But thinking about those things has become so much a part of my identity—I couldn't recognize myself in a certain kind of way." Anastasia said that it was "liberating to feel so functional," but the change was too much. She told her therapist that being able to at least *empathize* with someone with depression was important to her, and she asked to be put on a different drug. The medications she is on now, she said, strike the balance she needs; they let her feel "pretty much myself but just less, the really thin-skinned-ness or the kind of—I think without medication I feel almost too sensitive to live in the world. And I feel that with these things I'm a little protected from the world, but not so covered up that I feel nonhuman."

———

IN THIS CHAPTER, I told the stories of people who went from feeling lukewarm or worse about using medication, to feeling confident and comfortable with the role that it plays in their lives. In the beginning, James, Denise, and Anastasia felt as if they weren't in control of their choices around medication, and the associations it carried for them were mostly negative. James, as a teenager, was afraid of being judged by other people; to him, taking Prozac symbolized being crazy. Denise wasn't happy with how her G.P. handled her, didn't feel well listened to, and wasn't sure that the antidepressant he gave her really helped. Anastasia resented the sense that she had to use Zoloft to handle a job that she hated in the first place.

Then something happened to each that made them reevaluate their situation. James had another suicide attempt. Denise, shaken by her breakup, decided she'd been minimizing her dark feelings for long enough. Anastasia left the job she'd hated, but her depression didn't improve, it got worse. Each person made a return to medication and had a markedly better experience the second time around. They sought stronger relationships with doctors and found more effective drugs. They also began to assign more hopeful meanings to medication and to feel personally in charge of their decisions to use them. James began to see medication as, potentially, not just a palliative but also a key to the life he wanted; this committed him to keep searching for the right drugs, even when the search proved difficult. To Denise and Anastasia, medication started to symbolize a personal determination to take good care of themselves in a sometimes bruising world.

As I thought about the stories of James, Denise, and Anastasia—and also Dan from chapter 7—I found myself being guided to a theory. I don't think it's a coincidence that they all arrived at a feeling of greater security and greater positivity about their relationships with antidepressants as they moved into the second half of their twenties. In the last chapter, I wrote about how people who decided to stop using medication often felt that being a little older had made them more stable. But James, Denise, and Anastasia were also talking about the benefits of age. As I listened to their stories, it struck me that the existential worries that are front and center in younger people's antidepressant tales—the fears that medication might change their inmost natures—are no longer a major presence. This makes sense. As we age, the questions of identity that are a constant in adolescence begin to lose their keening insistency, not because we find the one diamond-hard answer we think we've been looking for, but because we settle into an intuitive sense of ourselves. "The older you get, the more secure you become in who you are," said Rachel, twenty-eight, explaining that she feels less torn about taking Effexor now than she did when she started as a young teenager, "and the more empathy you have for yourself too, and the more acceptance and self-esteem. I don't know why, but it just happens that way, as your ego kind of coalesces."

An e-mail I received from a twenty-six-year-old teacher named Debbie perfectly summed up the several kinds of evolution that make people who continue on medication tend to feel more comfortable about the decision as they mature.

When I first started taking Zoloft, at thirteen, I oscillated between being appalled at the idea and really wanting to take them. I wanted to take them because I felt like it somehow removed the blame from me. On the other hand,

I was not super thrilled with the idea of needing to be on anything, and I was definitely concerned about the way in which it would change me. I'd been depressed for as long as I could remember, and when I first started Zoloft I didn't know what it would feel like, and if I would act differently. It was hard to imagine a me who was cheerful. I also found (or at least claimed to find) cheerfulness insipid and I mistrusted good weather and people who seemed happy. They felt really artificial, and I felt like I was being artificial as well by taking antidepressants. I worried that I was putting up a buffer between myself and the world, and that I was dulling all of the input (the fact that I read *Brave New World* when I was fourteen did not help this).

I feel a lot better about taking them now. I think this is partially that I'm (fortunately) significantly more mature than I was when I was thirteen, and also that I don't think about it as much anymore. I've been on and off antidepressants for the past thirteen (!) years, so it's pretty much a habit. I've also learned that unexpected people take antidepressants as well, so I feel less alone. What they really do is help me live a normal life; I've found that, unfortunately, I can barely function without medicine. When I'm off my medicine, I get home at the end of the day and lie on the couch in my pajamas and can't do anything, I just sob and eventually go to bed. At this point, I have a responsibility to my husband as well as my parents and younger brother to stay on my medicine, or it becomes really difficult to deal with me, and that's not fair to them. I've tried to go off medicine before, and over time I've accepted that I will be on *something* probably for the rest of my life. It's still always in my mind somewhere, but ultimately I think I'm quite grateful that there are options to help me live a fairly normal life.

In Debbie's story, as in the other stories in this chapter, the central drama has shifted from "Who am I?" to "What do I need?" Debbie's choice to use medication is leveraged by her knowledge that she doesn't function well without it, but she doesn't speak of a sense of being forced into something that she doesn't want to do. What she does describe is what so many people feel as they grow into their adult selves: a greater sense of knowledge about what she needs and wants, and a greater willingness to reach out and grab it—to insist on it for herself, with ever-lessening amounts of conflict or doubt.

10 | THE NEXT GENERATION

In an accelerated culture, fifteen years is a long time. And it had been, I realized last spring when a cream-colored envelope arrived in my mailbox to announce preparations for my class's tenth college reunion, nearly that long since my experience with antidepressants began.

I knew that a lot must have changed in the interim. My peers and I were at college during the first wave of the SSRI revolution. During our midteen years, antidepressants weren't everywhere, and then suddenly they were; a spike in the number of students diagnosed with ADHD began just as we were graduating. People born in the 1990s were raised in a very different world. They had never known a time before Prozac, could scarcely remember when advertisements for prescription medication hadn't peered out from bus shelters and blared from TV. Did psychiatric medication mean something different to this generation than it had to mine?

At around the time that the invitation to my own tenth reunion arrived in the mail, I had been feeling curious about what had changed on college campuses since I last set foot on one. My interest was piqued by two sensational-sounding but widely reported stories in the news. One story proclaimed a remarkable recent deterioration in the mental health levels of college students. A 2010 survey of incoming college freshmen found that the self-reported mental well-being of incoming freshmen had fallen to its lowest level in twenty-five years, since the survey began collecting that information.[1] Another major survey found that 46 percent of college students had "felt things were hopeless" at some point in the previous year, while 30 percent had felt "so depressed that it was difficult to function."[2] Almost 95 percent of college and university mental health center directors in a national poll said that the number of students with "serious mental health problems" was "a growing concern" on their campus.[3] School mental health staffs found themselves dealing with an unprecedented volume of requests, and also with far more emergencies.[4] The number of students using medication had risen too; the University of California reported in 2006 that one in four students who arrived to seek counseling within the U.C. system was already taking a psychotropic medication that they had been prescribed elsewhere—a finding in keeping, the university noted, with a "stark increase" in medication use among student bodies nationwide.[5]

The second story reported on a precipitous rise in the amount of academic stress faced by college students. Undergraduate admissions had grown more competitive across the board in the past decade, as the children of baby boomers formed a miniboom of their own. Today's students were applying to more schools, facing more rejection, and living their pre-college lives ever more attuned to the need to work hard enough to vie for available spots.[6] Once admitted, according to longtime educators, students seemed apt to approach college as though it were a professional job, rather than a time for exploration and experimentation. One college president lamented that the "moments of woolgathering, dreaming, improvisation" that were seen as part and parcel of a liberal arts education a generation ago had become a hard sell for today's brand of highly driven student.[7] Experts agreed that undergraduates were in a bigger hurry than ever before, expected by teachers, parents, and themselves to produce more work, of a higher quality, in the same finite amount of time. Sometimes the stress story was linked to the mental-illness story, under the implication that a new generation of youth raised on pills and pushed to succeed were literally working themselves sick.[8]

I wondered whether these stories were true. What role did medication play on campus now, and what did students' attitudes toward it augur for the future? College, of course, isn't the only environment where young people use medication; it takes place in high schools and middle schools, and among young adults who don't attend college as well as those who do. But college remains one of the places where medication use is most concentrated and visible. There is a grain of truth to the idea that the affluent families who aspire to send their kids to private colleges are especially enthusiastic consumers of psychiatric services. For me, the question possessed the lure of returning to a once-familiar place to see what had changed in my absence. I decided to investigate how people more than ten years younger than I am think and feel about medication by visiting a college whose size and orientation reminded me a little bit of my own.

MADRIANNE WONG IS a senior at Swarthmore College in Swarthmore, Pennsylvania, a small commuter town about half an hour from

Philadelphia. I met up with her one afternoon in the campus library, a structure whose wood and stone interior reminded me a little of Frank Lloyd Wright's prairie architecture. We located each other by text message, and she came and joined me in a comfortable newspaper reading room. She greeted me warmly, said she had just come back from a run, and then sank into the armchair opposite mine. Her black skirt, torn black tights, and chunky asymmetrical haircut provided a pleasantly punky counterpoint to her instantly friendly demeanor.

Madrianne was the codirector of a campus group that offers free peer counseling to students. I found her through an article that she and her fellow director, junior Jessica Schleider, had published in the *Daily Gazette*, Swarthmore's online newspaper. Madrianne and Jessica believe that mental health issues are a growing problem on campus. They think that these problems are exacerbated by stress and academic pressure. But they also blame what they describe as a pervasive ethic of self-presentation on campus—in their article they call it a "culture of silence"—which demands that students appear not to have any problems at all. "There's an ideal of having everything together," Madrianne elaborated for me. "And everything encompasses not just academics; it's also social life; it's also, at least here, social activism, and it's also about looking good."

Students do feel comfortable talking about stress, Madrianne said, but only in a heroic mode—it's okay to complain about how much work you have to do, if it's in the context of describing how you were able to pull everything off at the last minute. Other negative feelings don't get talked about at all. "Being at Swarthmore," she said, "there's just this expectation of mental strength and resilience." It's an expectation that makes students loath to admit to any vulnerabilities, insecurities, or bona fide mental problems, even with close friends. "If you're here," said Madrianne, "you must perform—otherwise, there's this running joke about who the admissions mistake is." She and Jessica blame the "culture of silence" at Swarthmore for making students' mental problems worse. "At some point or another," they wrote in their *Daily Gazette* article, "all Swatties face issues, large and small. We can't sleep; we fight with roommates; we break up and are broken up with. We worry for troubled friends. We feel overwhelmed, inadequate, or misunderstood; we experience depression, anxiety, and eating disorders. Most dangerously, we fear being judged for our struggling . . . as a result, we don't share, and we feel alone."[9]

Madrianne and Jessica weren't the first to point out a campus taboo against seeming anything short of perfect. In fact, they borrowed the phrase "culture of silence" from an article penned earlier that year by a Yale senior named Julia Lurie. In her piece, Lurie described Yale as a place in which mental problems were both ubiquitous and undiscussed. She wrote of laboring to turn herself into the Yale ideal, someone not just academically on top of things, but also popular, socially engaged, worldly, ambitious, involved in interesting and unique extracurriculars. Outwardly she had succeeded in transforming herself into the multipotent model student; she was the type of girl who "makes intelligent-sounding comments in seminar and the professor nods, but you can see she's checking her e-mail—you wonder how she's following the conversation." How surprised her classmates would be, she confessed, if they could see the other Julia Lurie, the one who was anything but effortless, the girl who "takes her Zoloft and a sleeping pill" each night, then "writhes in hot, silent tears, white-knuckled, feeling like she could scream."[10] The larger point of Lurie's piece was that emotional hypocrisy was endemic on campus: we all know nobody's perfect, but at Yale, no one will admit that they're not. As a result, people suffer in silence. She closed the article with a call for increased honesty and greater mental health awareness on campus.

Joseph Davis is a sociology professor at the University of Virginia. For several years he has been conducting a study of undergraduates' attitudes toward antidepressants and ADHD medications, interviewing dozens of students indepth about their use of these drugs. In his research, Davis has noticed a pattern similar to the one that Madrianne Wong and Julia Lurie describe, in which undergraduates at elite schools spoke of a need to seem "flawless." He talked to student after student who described feeling an urgent need to live up to their "full potential," a state that those students often conceived of in confusingly nebulous terms.[11] The students told Davis that they did not feel comfortable confiding their doubts and anxieties to their friends. Unsurprisingly, many of them were unaware that other students also experienced performance anxiety or felt dissatisfied with themselves.

Davis uses the term "the achieving self" to describe the ideal to which these students strive.[12] The achieving self possesses a number of impressive qualities that are hard enough to attain on their own, and sometimes actually contradict one another. "While proactive, aggressive, and impressive," he writes, "this self is also easy-going, nondefensive, flexible, resilient, and resourceful."[13] Davis believes that some students use psychiatric medication partly in an attempt to conform to the demands of the achieving self, including its prohibition against the expression of negative feelings including "discouragement and loneliness, nervousness and insecurity, jealousy and emotional vulnerability, shame and humiliation, regret and self-blame."[14] A Swarthmore student named Michelle, who uses antidepressants, put the same thought to me in a different way. When I asked her whether she felt that there was a stigma on campus attached to taking medication, she replied, "I don't feel like the stigma is necessarily against the drug aspect of it. The stigma is just against feeling bad. Because if you're on drugs, but you seem to be totally fine, then whatever. My roommate is also on a medication for anxiety, and we talk about it very cavalierly—like, 'Oh yeah, I'm going to take my meds now; I'll go crazy if I don't, ha ha.' It's just kind of tossed around. And I've heard that happening with other people too, not just my close friends. So there definitely is a pressure to sort of be perfectly competent in everything, but it has a weird relationship with the antidepressant aspect of it."

Madrianne, Jessica, Julia Lurie, and Joseph Davis all describe a world in which medications are thought of not necessarily as treating well-defined mental illnesses, but are seen as a way of easing pressure and of saving face in a public environment that demands a smooth self-presentation. Jessica Schleider told me that she believes a lot of people take medication almost prophylactically, to ensure that they're able to perform up to their own highest standards. "The way [medications] are seen on campus is like, 'If I'm taking them, then I'll be fine,'" she said. "'Now I'll be on top of things. Now I'll have no excuse.'"

Though students don't often talk to one another about their vulnerabilities, Madrianne and Jessica gain a unique vantage point through their work as peer counselors. Madrianne told me that students often say they're confused about whether any given feeling they're having is a sign of illness, and whether or not they need or would benefit from medication. In a world where everyone else puts on a perfect face, it's difficult or impossible to know when your own bad feelings cross over the line from normal to abnormal. "People are always wondering whether they're experiencing something they shouldn't be," she said, "or if the way they are feeling is wrong." She told me that one of the questions students ask her most frequently is whether or not they should go to counseling services and "get a label"—be diagnosed and possibly get a prescription for the problem. Jessica also noted that she's observed students feeling unsure about diagnosis and medication. "Nobody sleeps in college, right?" she said. "Everyone's stressed-out. Everyone gets sad. And everyone knows that drugs are an option. So it's just confusing to people. Like, 'Should I really pursue this? Am I sick enough for this? Am I sick at all? Is this really what sick is?'"

MANY OF THE students who wonder whether or not they need a mental health diagnosis end up in the office of David Ramirez, director of Swarthmore's Counseling and Psychological Services, or CAPS. I met Ramirez in the building that houses the counseling center, a large stone cottage with a peaked roof; his office was spacious but cluttered with a pleasantly random assortment of institutional upholstered furniture. Ramirez, who has been the director of CAPS for seventeen years, has short black hair that is flecked with a little gray. He wore two-tone plastic glasses, a fleece vest, and black hiking boots; before he worked in college mental health, he told me, he used to lead outdoor trips for emotionally disturbed middle school students. It was spring break, the first time all semester that Ramirez had had a free moment:

CAPS, for reasons he didn't completely understand, had been overwhelmed for months. "It's freaky, actually," he said.

I asked Ramirez whether there'd really been an upsurge in the amount of mental illness on campus, and he said there had. "There's no doubt about that," he said. "It's a cultural phenomenon." The college years have always been a period when a number of mental illnesses often manifest for the first time; it's a classic age for the first psychotic breaks of schizophrenia or bipolar disorder. But Ramirez believes that serious issues are truly on the rise: "The number of people and the intensity of problems have both increased over time," he said. Past suicide attempts, he told me, are a gauge; over the years, he's seen more and more students who made previous attempts on their own lives, as high school, middle school, or even elementary school students. Some experts believe that at least part of the perceived increase in mental illness on college campuses is due to a hopeful trend—a product of the fact that more vigorous treatment has meant that kids who once might not have been able to go away to college can now leave home and attend the school of their choice.

Like other college mental health center directors I spoke to, Ramirez also agreed that academic stress has increased over time. Madrianne and a couple of other students had already told me stories about how little they sleep—a seemingly even-keeled senior averred that he made it through his first three years at Swarthmore on about four hours a night—and Ramirez added that if he could make one intervention on campus to better the mental health of all, he'd choose improved "sleep hygiene" in a heartbeat. Gary Margolis, who has headed the counseling center at Middlebury College for thirty-eight years, said he'd absolutely watched the demands on the quality and quantity of student academic work and extracurricular engagement increase during his career. Nor have the changes been confined to elite institutions. A school counselor at a tier-two regional university told me much the same thing. "There does seem to be a lot more pressure than there was even when I was in school [ten to fifteen years ago]," she said. "It feels like the rat race has sped up."

While he acknowledges the stress that students are under, Ramirez cautioned that it would be a mistake to make a simple equation between increased pressure on campus and increased mental illness. Stress doesn't cause serious mental disorder, and removing a mentally ill person from a stressful environment won't make their illness go away. That said, Ramirez believes that stress exacerbates mental health problems on campus, intensifying the distress that students do feel, and influencing the kind of help that they decide to seek.

For one thing, he noted, stress contributes to a pervasive feeling of urgency, so that students who feel bad are in an extreme hurry to feel better. This can mean that students who come to CAPS feel motivated to get a prescription for a medication, because they perceive it as the fastest way to recover. Other counseling center directors I talked to noted the same shift. "When a student's upset, they're upset in the moment," said Vivien Chan, chief of mental health services at U.C. Irvine. "It's very dissatisfying to tell a student to come back tomorrow, or wait two weeks. Because two weeks to a college student, that's a lifetime." Gary Margolis of Middlebury added that "students come to counseling expecting that something quick is going to happen that's going to change how they feel." He said that a preference for medication over counseling is often conditioned by the fact that students don't feel like they can afford the loss of engagement from their work or activities that might occur while they wait for talk therapy to make a difference. Taking time to process feelings has come to seem like a quaint notion, an indulgence as outdated as nine hours of sleep or a just-for-fun elective. Even Madrianne, who does not use antidepressants and feels ambivalent about diagnostic labeling, snorted at the labor-intensive approach that campus counseling centers were once known for. "The amount of time you spend in counseling—who has that much time?" she said. "Finding an hour to have lunch with someone, it's—I mean, there's a bunch of points against getting help that isn't a quick fix."

Second, said Ramirez, students are often understandably confused about what's pathological. Mental disorder is a convenient, available explanation for all kinds of trouble, and he often sees students reaching for it, or accepting it when it is suggested to them. Such suggestions are everywhere. Students have family members and friends who use medications. They are exposed to on-campus screening days for depression and other mental disorders, events that are often sponsored by pharmaceutical companies.[15] They hear stories about ancestors who were considered to be 'crazy'; knowing that mental illness runs in families, they worry that it's going to happen to them. Often a student will come to Ramirez because someone else has labeled them. "I can't tell you the number of people who come in because someone's told them they have ADD," he said. "Because, what? Yes, they have attention and concentration problems. But they haven't slept in a week!" All of these examples are signs of a broader cultural shift that has blurred the line between mental illness and the baseline quotient of sadness, anxiety, and stress that into each life must fall. "Things that we didn't used to think of as being psychiatric disorders are now considered to be psychiatric problems," Ramirez said. "There's been kind of a pathologization of life itself."

All in all, Ramirez told me, students haven't changed since he first got into the field. Throughout his two decades in school counseling, students have presented with a remarkably stable set of cares. "The concerns that people have—'Am I going to be loved? Am I going to be successful? What's life all about?'"—these, Ramirez says, are the questions that students have always asked, in their million different ways. What's different today is that students are much more likely to attach these questions, and their worries around them, to the idea of diagnosable mental illness.

I told Ramirez about something I'd been mulling over since reading Julia Lurie, Madrianne, and Jessica's articles. It had struck me that students are very able to talk about "stress," and very able to talk about "mental health issues" (even if it's in the context of bemoaning low awareness), but that there didn't seem to be much conversation about negative feelings outside of the rubric of mental health. I had been surprised to find what I would consider "ordinary" feelings lumped in with clinical mental problems: in Madrianne and Jessica's article, depression, anxiety, and eating disorders were name-checked as "mental health issues," but so were insomnia, fights with roommates, romantic breakups, and the sensation of being misunderstood. Ramirez agreed. In the context of a culture where many of the "baseline phenomena" of life have come to be considered symptoms of illness, he said, there's a lot of confusion about what is and isn't acceptable to feel. "Young people aren't sure how to think about their distress," he said. "There's almost not a language for normal distress."

The loss of a vocabulary for normal distress is accompanied by a loss of perspective. Much of what Ramirez says he does as a counselor is to try to help students think through what the stressors in their lives are, to try to figure out for themselves the boundary between understandable amounts of strife and real pathology. "We try to contextualize it," he said. Plenty of times, it will turn out that students were laboring under burdens they hadn't really considered before. "Sometimes you get someone saying 'Yeah, now that I think of it, my favorite grandfather *did* just die, and I didn't get to go home for the funeral.' Just terrible things, that if the pace of their life doesn't allow for the integration of these experiences, then it's a problem." If a student's feelings appear to be in a normal range, says Ramirez, "we ask, 'considering all these things that are depressing you, what is your expectation of how you *should* be feeling right now?'"

Learning why you feel the way you feel is a skill that has to be acquired. Most students don't come to college with an advanced understanding of the forces at work on them. "If you could do some kind of regression analysis of lines that people have said in counseling," Ramirez said, "probably one of the most frequently uttered phrases would be something like, 'I don't know what's wrong with me; I have everything a person could want in life, and I'm still depressed.'" Many psychiatrists would take such a statement at face value—feeling bad without reason equals depression—but Ramirez thinks it's more complicated than that. Especially at a school like Swarthmore, students are often conscious of their own privilege. They've been groomed all their lives for college, and they may have no idea why they suddenly feel let down or lost. Ramirez thinks there are plenty of reasons, up to and including the enormous value placed on getting into a good school, but says that students looking for an explanation are often inclined to find it in the idea of a mood disorder or other inner problem.

RAMIREZ'S COMMENT ABOUT a regression analysis immediately brought to mind my interview with Caitlin. Caitlin attends a large private university in the Northeast. She is nineteen years old and a sophomore. On the phone, she sounded perky, warm, and agreeable. She described herself as "really outgoing" and mentioned that she was involved in a lot of activities at school: she gave campus tours, worked an additional job at the library coffee shop, belonged to a service fraternity, and headed up the school's chapter of UNICEF. She was on the go from 9:00 A.M. to 10:00 P.M. or later every day, she said, and that's the way she liked it. She told me that she's not the kind of person anyone expects to have depression. "The couple people I have told, it throws them off," she said.

College started well for Caitlin. "I made some good friends," she said. "I was getting involved in a ton of stuff. I was happy with how everything was going. I even liked my classes." She told me that she had been looking forward to college for a long time, not least because it meant an opportunity to get away from home. "My mom and I really don't get along," Caitlin said. "So in high school, I'd be fine at school, I'd be fine with my friends, and then I'd come home. And it was whenever I came in contact with my mom, I started having, I called them 'dark spirals.' I would start to feel a depression whenever I was around her." She was eager to get to college because she expected that getting out of the house would bring her dark spirals to an end.

But at college, though Caitlin was often happy, sometimes

her mood would deteriorate and "it all just felt like shit." I asked her why, and she replied, in words much like the ones David Ramirez had described hearing from his students, "I think that's kind of what the issue was. I *should* have been happy." She had been counting on distance from her mother to make things better, and she felt worried and discouraged that it hadn't completely worked. "It was hard to handle the fact that it wasn't just my mom, and I couldn't just remove myself from the situation, but rather there was something bigger or worse," Caitlin said. In college, during the bad times, Caitlin could imagine hurting herself in some way, and even though "I knew that I really wasn't going to," the thoughts were disturbing.

Toward the end of her first year, Caitlin said, "I remember there was one day when I decided to go [to the psychiatrist]. I had, like, an emotional breakdown. It was the end of my freshman year in college, right at the end of the year, getting ready to go home. And for some reason I just had a really rough night. I was sitting on the edge of my bed, and bawling my eyes out. Just sitting there thinking, 'There's nothing wrong with my life, so why am I feeling like this?'"

Back at home, Caitlin sought out a psychiatrist who gave her a prescription for an antidepressant. When we talked, she had been on it for about six months. She told me she thought the medication was helping, but she didn't sound entirely sure. "I mean, I definitely can notice it," she said. "So I think it's working. But who knows?" She told me she didn't especially enjoy taking medication, and that she hopes she won't have to continue forever.

What struck me about Caitlin's story was how many things she did have to feel bad about, even if she didn't recognize them.

She had conflict with her mother. As the youngest child of the family, she felt that both of her parents babied her. She wanted to let them know that she was her own person now, but she also confessed that she "hates confrontation," so she was having a hard time figuring out how to express her feelings of independence. She was experimenting with abandoning her parents' Catholic faith but didn't feel she could tell them about that either. She was tremendously busy with school. And she was dealing with the developmental and separation tasks that all college students must deal with. The fact that those tasks are ubiquitous doesn't make them any less daunting. Gertrude Carter, a psychologist who headed the student mental health service at Bennington College for many years, told me she believes that most college students are in a state of grief when they arrive at college, or fall into one soon after. "No matter what, there are losses," she said. "You leave your friends, you leave your family. You're on your own in a completely alien environment, and it's supposed to be just wonderful, but it often isn't." The challenge of this dislocation seems obvious to me now, as an older person, but I remember being as blind to it then as Caitlin seemed to be.

I thought that it made sense for Caitlin's distress to come to a head on the eve of her return home for the summer, but that's not how she saw it. It was clear that seeing a psychiatrist had been a way for her to take herself seriously and express the independence that she craved from her parents, who she said did not approve of her decision to take medication. But like the students Ramirez described, she didn't have a language for normal distress. In fact, the explanation Caitlin gave of how she was able to feel happy one moment and depressed the next was that "for me, maybe there's some bipolar thing in there too."

IF ANTIDEPRESSANTS ARE helping to blur the distinction between ordinary and pathological feelings on college campuses, so are the psychostimulant medications that are prescribed for ADHD. Their use as study drugs has grabbed a lot of headlines in recent years: a dose will allow you to stay up all night, keeping your eyes glued to your books, while you write that long-procrastinated paper. Though it is hard to track exactly, says Vivien Chan of U.C. Irvine, misuse of prescription stimulants on college campuses is rampant. Students, she said, describe acquiring these drugs as "effortless"; the library is often a hot spot for sales, though it's likely that most students don't have to go much farther than a few doors down their dormitory hallway.

Chan told me that the abuse of Adderall and other psycho-stimulants is at least partly due to legitimate confusion on the part of students about what constitutes a normal ability to focus. "I think college is tough," she said. "The students are under tremendous pressure. Almost all of them feel like they could be studying better, or studying more. It's really easy for everybody to be worried about keeping up and paying attention. Of a hundred students who walk into my clinic, if you ask them whether they have problems with concentration, 99 percent of them are going to say yes." At Irvine, she sees a steady stream of students who confide in her that they somehow obtained an Adderall pill, that it really helped them, and by the way, they've always kind of had trouble concentrating, and does she think they might have ADHD? Chan gently tries to tell students whom she believes don't need stimulants that they aren't necessary. But she concedes that the call can be a difficult one to make, since like all mental disorders, there's no objective test for ADHD.

Kristin, twenty-two, who graduated last year from a university in the South, takes Adderall on her doctor's orders and believes that she needs it—but in general, she said, she sees school stress playing into people's decisions to use pharmaceuticals, both prescribed and diverted. She believes that some people turn to medication to deal with problems that might be manageable in other ways, if not for the pace and pressure of school. "I don't know how many people are on [medication] because they really need it," she said. "But it's easy for the doctor to say 'Why don't we put you on this and see how you do.' Because when you're in college, you can't stop and figure things out. I think that a lot of people, in terms of personal physical and mental health, should take a break between years of college." But that isn't always possible, and medication can help students endure. Now that she's graduated, Kristin explained, "I definitely feel far less anxiety just not having any school to deal with." Work and social stress, she said, are easy in comparison. When I asked her what made academic stress different, she exclaimed, "Everyone tells you that school's going to determine the rest of your life! It just starts to build up after a while."

Small colleges aren't the only places where students are confused about how they ought to feel, and look to medication as a way to function as highly as they think they should. The week after I visited Swarthmore, I stopped in to see a psychiatrist who works in a private practice in Manhattan, and treats many college students and recent grads. "I feel like the expectations that a lot of patients have seem to be unrealistic," she said,

in the sense of "I should be able to work fourteen hours a day, and then go out and have a social life, and maintain a certain weight, and not be exhausted." The number of people who come in here and tell me that they don't sleep well or they never have enough energy, and then when you review what their day is like—there seems to be a disconnect between [what they expect and] what is possible, what one can possibly do in a day. There's a sense that they're turning to pharmaceuticals to make something possible that's not healthy or normal.

She added that she often felt surprised by how little sense the young adults she sees have of what constitute normal, healthy routines, or of the way they can expect their behavior to influence how they feel. "A lot of [street] drug use has become so normalized that many people don't understand that if you are severely depressed and you have trouble functioning already, that smoking pot all day long is not going to help that," she said. She is alarmed by the number of students who think they ought to be able to work all day every day, party each night, and still feel okay—and who define their inability to do that as a problem to be solved through medication. "It's surprising to me the things that people come in to talk to me about," she mused. "A lot of it is issues that, if people had internalized more normal routines earlier in life—I mean, do you really need me to tell you that you should be sleeping seven hours a night? That you should eat three times a day?"

Without a doubt, the SSRI revolution has brought about some positive changes on campuses. Gary Margolis of Middlebury pointed out to me that in the 1960s, before colleges generally had counseling centers of any kind, students with mental or emotional problems had little choice but to "suffer silently," self-medicate with alcohol, drugs, or food, or withdraw from school. "Some of those students disappeared, literally," he said. "I can remember classmates who were present, and then all of a sudden you realized that they weren't in the dorm, they weren't in class. They had withdrawn, without any explanation."

But it's clear that the increase in medication use at colleges reflects more than just a surge in cases of serious mental illness. A portion of the rise is guided by factors that Madrianne Wong and Jessica Schleider were well aware of: an environment in which, because of a variety of factors converging—from a national context where emotions once regarded as everyday nuisances are now seen as signs of disease, to a local context where students don't share with one another their negative feelings and thus come to believe that they're alone in them, to a high-pressure academic climate that can exacerbate medium-size problems into big ones and prevent students from taking the time to reflect and integrate—students become inclined to interpret their distress as a mental disorder, and to reach out for medication or have medication suggested to them as the cure.

AND WELL, YOU might ask, so what? If these medications are safe—and they're fairly safe—and if they make the stressful life of a college student easier to bear, then what's the harm?

I can think of a few places to look. The first is back to the idea of a "culture of silence." Keeping quiet with peers enforces unrealistic expectations, in a kind of feedback loop: students who can't share their doubts and insecurities don't know that other students also feel bad, so they assume that their own bad feelings must be abnormal, which makes those feelings worse and harder to open up about. Inasmuch as psychiatric drug use helps students to live up to the mandates of the "achieving self," it also helps to keep the culture of silence strong and in place, and may preclude conversations that could lead to more realistic expectations about feelings and accomplishments. (Madrianne Wong, Jessica Schleider, and Julia Lurie called for greater "mental health awareness" to address the culture of silence, but I wasn't sure their impulse was exactly the right one. Awareness is important, but it seems to me that it's precisely the tendency to define all emotional difficulties as "signs of mental disorder" that makes it harder for students to share their feelings and to experience the resulting sense of camaraderie.)

Second, medications can harm if the hurried approach to recovery that they represent discourages students from taking a deeper look at what's wrong. Away from the routines defined by home and family, college students must start to explore the way that the choices they make in their personal lives, and the care they take of their bodies, make them feel. But the view that comes along with medication— that many negative feelings and physical limitations are symptoms of illness—can discourage students from learning how to make these connections and deprive them of a chance to discover more autonomous or creative ways of dealing with their problems. Gertrude Carter of Bennington and her staff psychiatrist, Jeffrey Winseman, made just that point in a 2001 article in the *Chronicle of Higher Education*. They were troubled by the stream of students coming through their office doors who already took medication habitually; many had had their prescriptions renewed for years on end without complaint. Carter and Winseman weren't against medication as part of a thoughtful treatment plan, but they were highly critical of the "medication only" approach they saw signs of. "If we respond to our students' pain in purely biological terms," they wrote, "we exclude the potential for change through the understanding of meaningful experiences."

Third, psychiatric medication teaches students to look for the source of their pain inside of themselves, not in the world they live in. Joseph Davis believes that much of the distress that students suffer is produced by their environment—specifically, by the notable increase in pressure to perform that has affected college, high school, and even elementary school students in recent decades. In his research, he has found that students are seldom aware of the forces that operate on them, and that students who use medication are especially likely to define their problems as unique and arising from within. "There's a tendency to take on any kind of failure or problem as though there's something wrong with you, that you're broken or something like that," he said. "Student after student would come in [to be interviewed], saying almost identical things, but then attribute it to 'there's something wrong with me,' or 'this is just something of mine, I was born this way.' And you wished they could hear each other talking."

Davis knows, from the times he's presented his research to young audiences, how reassuring students find it to learn that they're not alone in their feelings, and that some of their anxieties might be situational and not just innate. "I think it does give people more of a sense of agency," he said. "If you know you're under certain kinds of pressures, you may be able to address them more directly, or feel less threatened by them." If someone feels bad for a reason, it doesn't seem right or even particularly helpful to inform them that they are suffering from a chemical imbalance. It might even be socially conservative. As the cultural critic Matthew Crawford wrote recently, tracing all psychic unease back to individual biology "seems to neutralize any impulse to criticize the world"—and such criticism, after all, can be considered one main goal of a liberal education.[16]

Finally, the question of criticizing the world, or the wisdom of locating the problem in one's environment versus locating the problem in oneself, is especially important in light of the fact that a majority of the young people who use antidepressants are girls. It's no accident that a majority of the examples in this chapter—and in this book—have been female. In childhood, boys' and girls' rates of depression are comparable, but around age twelve or thirteen, girls surge ahead; for the rest of the life span, women experience about twice as much depression as men.[17]

There are many theories to explain why this might be, and some of the strong ones are social. Researchers and psychologists have pegged the higher rate of girls' and womens' depression to everything from greater incidence of childhood sexual abuse,[18] to a culture that encourages girls and women to be polite and "nice" all the time and squelch expressions of anger and aggression. (It is certainly interesting that the great self-squelching project documented by psychologists like Carol Gilligan, Lyn Mikel Brown, and Mary Pipher occurs during the junior high years,[19] the same time when girls' rates of depression begin their upward climb.) Another factor is the prevalence of eating disorders and body-image problems among girls and young women (studies show that up to 64 percent of college women display disordered eating patterns,[20] and I was struck that a majority of the college-aged women I spoke to mentioned body image as a significant psychological stressor). In 2011, a UCLA researcher named Linda Sax found that there is a gender gap in self-reported mental well-being among incoming college freshmen, with female students claiming lower levels of mental wellness than male ones; Sax found that this gap has actually been growing larger over the last twenty-five years.[21] Though college women earn better grades and graduate at higher rates than their male counterparts, they consistently estimate their academic abilities lower than men do, and the difference in confidence between men and women increases during college.[22]

Young women who are depressed, for any reason, need help and care. But if girls suffer psychologically in part because they try hard to be perfect and pleasant, learning to hide their feelings of anger and sadness even from themselves, then a culture in which we "treat" young women's sadness by telling them that it's a disorder that arises from within their own minds seems likely to reinforce these harmful dynamics, not fix them. Psychiatry has a long, unfortunate history of pathologizing women. The SSRI era, with its stated commitment to science, carried at least an implicit promise that old, sexist categories like "hysteria" would be left behind in favor of a more empirical approach. We need to remain vigilant to the possibility that the transformation hasn't been complete, partly by not being too quick to hand girls a cure that reduces their suffering to native craziness.[23] Young women deserve good treatment. But the best treatment will not discourage them from thinking critically about the extraordinary, changing, sometimes conflicting expectations that shape the experience of modern womanhood, and the ways that these expectations fit into the larger picture of mental health.

BEFORE GETTING IN my rental car for the drive back to New York, I spent a while walking around the Swarthmore campus. It was dark by then, and clear, with a moon. The grounds seemed quiet without students, but here and there I heard voices, a snatch of laughter. Light and music drifted out of the second-story window of a stone dorm. By any measure, it was a beautiful place. But like all campuses, it was part of the world and fully permeable to its problems.

I thought that it would be nice to imagine a world in which the pressures on college students would slacken—where students would feel as though they had enough time to get a good night's sleep, or spend a couple weeks weathering a breakup or a fight in the expectation that the feelings would fade over time. I wished that students could better understand the structures that condition their lives, but I saw that even if that were possible, they might not be able to do much with the knowledge. Medications do fill a need, and it seems only reasonable to assume that they'll keep on filling it.

And maybe that doesn't need to be a catastrophe. I've spoken about the tyranny of perfectionism and the ways in which medication can enforce it, both for individuals and communities. But it doesn't have to. As I walked, I thought back to my own conversation earlier that day with Nicole, a Swarthmore student I sat with over coffee, beside the plate glass windows of the new science center near the back of campus. Nicole was her own kind of perfect girl, in an intellectual Swarthmore mode. She was an honors student at work on her biochemistry thesis; she played music in a chamber group, spent the summer doing original research at an oceanographic laboratory in California, took the train to Philadelphia to attend genetics grand rounds at the children's hospital, and was involved in a couple of campus groups.

She told me she had wanted to do medical research since she was in the third grade. After graduation, she would begin applying to MD/PhD programs in her field.

Nicole's antidepressant story began the summer after her freshman year. She went through a bad breakup and spent the end of the season crying and too anxious to eat. The next semester she struggled in classes, developed a stomach problem, and got cut from the varsity soccer team.

Her mother took her to a psychiatrist back home in Minnesota over winter break. The psychiatrist put her on Lexapro. "It was a relief to be diagnosed," Nicole said. "I had a lot of pressure on myself to achieve, and when I failed my standards, I got really ripped up about it, and I just thought that I was a failure. So when I got diagnosed, all I could think was, 'It's not my fault.'"

Nicole went to CAPS once for counseling but says that, as someone who's interested in biological medicine, "I didn't really know if counseling was going to make a difference. And I'm afraid my skepticism may have communicated itself to my counselor. She actually told me that she felt uncomfortable because she felt like I was judging her. Anyway, I didn't get a lot out of it." She never went back.

She did find the Lexapro helpful. The medication "gave me a floor," Nicole said, "where my emotions couldn't go lower than that." On the other hand, she "took myself off" Lexapro after five months because she felt it was negatively impacting her academic performance. "I decided that it was making me gray out, like apathy. I just didn't care if I got my work in on time." But by that point, her life had stabilized, and she felt as though the worst of the depression had gone. She says that she's glad to be off medication, but she's deeply grateful that it was there for her when she needed it. "I only wish it had been caught earlier," she says of her depression, using the biomedical language that she prefers.

Nicole ascribed wholeheartedly to the biochemical interpretation of depression, but she didn't see that view as an invitation not to explore the way the world, or her choices in it, makes her feel. If anything, it's the opposite: because she is prone to depression, Nicole said, she has to be vigilant and take good care of herself. "I employ a lot of strategies to make sure that the depression doesn't come back," she told me. She described surrounding herself with positive people, monitoring her own thought patterns, and making sure she spends enough social time with her chamber group. "I think isolation is a huge component" of depression, she said. "A lot of us are introverts, and it's easy to hide in your room."

Nicole spoke of her depression and treatment as a learning experience. In particular, she said, it helped her gain some perspective on the culture of perfection and her own expectations of herself. In addition to making her take her own needs more seriously, her experience with depression helped her to see through the bright and shining myth of the perfect student. "Everyone's so ambitious when they get here," she told me. "They think they can do everything. And the college says 'Yeah, you can do everything!' But you can't." Still highly driven today, Nicole said that now she understands the difference between excellence, which is real, and flawlessness, which can't be. "Until I fell apart and put myself together I could not accept that being good at something was enough," she said. "I had to be the best. And you can never be the best. Not without falling apart."

In the mid-2000s, the Pfizer corporation ran a major print and television advertising campaign for Zoloft. The concept was a bit avant-garde for a pharmaceutical product. Instead of human actors, the ads featured cartoons. The main character was a crudely drawn oval, white with a rough black outline, that most viewers referred to as a "ball" or an "egg." At the beginning of each TV commercial, the ball suffered pathetically—cowering in a corner with social anxiety disorder, or languishing under a dark cloud of depression. By the end, successfully treated with antidepressants, the ball smiled and bounced, joining a room full of fellow balls celebrating in party hats, or horsing around playfully with its friends, a red ladybug and a blue butterfly.

In fact, the series was brilliant. Using a cartoon character represented a stroke of genius; somehow the abstract blob swept away the resistance it's so easy to feel when watching live actors. "I just want the sad, badly drawn circle to regain its happiness," read a typical comment in an online forum. "I feel more empathy and goodwill toward it than to the legion of live actors in various commercials. Kind of strange, really." The simplicity of the ball character—just a circular line with two eyes and a mouth—belied an incredible expressiveness. It *was* kind of strange how easy it was to get emotionally involved with the little guy. It was also hard to watch the commercials without wondering, at least for a moment, whether you could use some Zoloft yourself; the distance from emotional involvement to identification, and from identification to imagining how the product might make you feel, was just two brief hops.

When I search for a way to describe the change antidepressants have brought about during my generation, I think of what's communicated in these commercials. To live in America today is to be invited, again and again, to ask ourselves whether our problems are symptoms, to consider whether we need or would simply benefit from a psychiatric medication. For some people, antidepressants are more legitimately considered a need than an option. But for millions of others who occupy the large middle ground between definitely requiring medication and definitely not, antidepressants exist as a possibility: available and acceptable, they are always on the table, a potential we remain well aware of, whether we use them or not. Access to medication is controlled by physicians, but the urging to "ask your doctor" is commercial and omnipresent. In a very real sense, medication has become a consumer choice, just one more in the ocean of such choices that define our modern lives.

Certainly there's much to celebrate about the antidepressant option. Placebo or not, the medications work, alleviating serious depression, "mere" sadness and borderline states alike. People who are grateful for their medication number in the millions. Among the antidepressant users and former users I talked to, even those who felt ambivalent about antidepressants often expressed appreciation that they exist. There's a small fortitude that comes from simply knowing that there's help available, something we could try if we wanted to.

But while having the choice to use antidepressants represents freedom, it also brings a type of anxiety all its own. Social psychologists have repeatedly shown that despite the advantages they confer, proliferating options sap decision-making energy and multiply the possibilities for regret.[1] Medication is no exception. My peers and I have gained the power of being able to change how we feel, but we have also had to assume the necessity of wondering, at any point, whether we are choosing correctly. To medicate, or not to medicate? This question, with its accompanying undertow of slight worry, has become part of the atmosphere. To live in the age of SSRIs is to know that there are possibilities, and to have to choose one mode of living over another. It's hard not to wonder whether there's something about the road not taken that would have been better, or even to feel that either path leaves something to be desired. We exist in the bind that Carl Elliott's work on authenticity pointed to: shall we be happy but unnatural, or natural but less than perfectly happy?

As the use of psychiatric medication becomes more prevalent in children and younger teens, the anxiety of choice around medication is increasingly transferred onto parents. In the course of my research for this book, I spoke to several parents who approached the decision to place their kids on medication surefootedly, without much doubt about which course of action their situation demanded. But others described a deep and lasting uncertainty. "The sense of parental guilt is enormous," said a father, fifty, who had considered antidepressants for his teenage son and ADHD medication for his younger daughter, after a school friend's parents and a teacher suggested that the children might benefit. He and his wife eventually decided against medication for both of their children, but they still felt haunted by the choice, and they revisited it occasionally. A mother of three in the Midwest told me that her debate with her husband about whether to start their precocious five-year-old on Ritalin was the fiercest conflict they had faced in their marriage to date. She too reported feeling condemned to a sense of guilt no matter what she chose: she could keep her son off medication and worry about denying him something that he might need or gain from, or she could place him on medication and worry about interfering with his natural development. Both possibilities seemed equally frightening; when we spoke, she had recently agreed to a trial period on Ritalin for her son, but she reported feeling far from peaceful about the choice.

Despite the existence of experts to help parents face these decisions, the call often feels frustratingly subjective. To some extent, it is: there are still no objective or physical tests for mental disorder. Indeed, as the bioethicists Erik Parens and Josephine Johnston point out, the question of whether or not to medicate children and adolescents who are not severely ill can legitimately be considered a question of values. Reasonable people, including doctors, can and do disagree about where to draw the line between normal and abnormal feelings in kids and teenagers, and they disagree about how to weigh the advantages and disadvantages of medicating.[2] In the end, the burden of this uncertainty falls on parents, who find that they must face the choice of whether to use medication, and hold the possibility of making a mistake, on their own.

It is ironic that medication has become a choice that we're perennially hovering over. Despite the DSM task force's "increased commitment to reliance on data as the basis for understanding mental disorders," the last twenty years have seen an increase both in our collective confusion about what mental illness is and about where the boundaries of normal should be drawn. Diagnostic brackets creep, as Peter Kramer said once. As our vocabulary for sadness, conflict, alienation, and exhaustion merges with the language of biomedical mental disorder, we lose the language of ordinary distress. The nonmedical words come to seem imprecise or old-fashioned. As it spreads, the new language breeds uncertainty, until almost any uncomfortable feeling comes to seem potentially abnormal. In our age, it has become increasingly hard to feel sad, angry, or overwhelmed—or have someone close to you feel that way—without wondering if you, or they, are sick. While no doubt there remain places in this country where mental health care is still badly underdelivered, in the pockets where awareness reigns, we crossed over some time ago into what a psychologist would call a state of hypervigilance.

Maybe some part of this puzzlement about normalcy is old, just the latest vestige of a long-standing anxiety about how we ought to feel. The question of how much happiness we should feel and express has been an active one in America for centuries, with different answers prevailing in different times and contexts. Perhaps the question seems written into our Declaration of Independence itself: maybe there has always been slippage in our minds between the idea of a right to pursue happiness, and a duty to *be* happy, a sense that if we aren't sucking the marrow out of life, aren't using our extraordinary freedom to its greatest advantage at all times, we aren't, somehow, fulfilling our job as Americans.

Whatever its causes, the extraordinary proliferation of

psychiatric drug use that began twenty-five years ago with the arrival of Prozac shows few signs of slowing. Spending on prescription drugs in the United States more than doubled between 1999 and 2008, thanks in part to sales of psychopharmaceuticals.[3] As of 2009, 9 percent of five-to-seventeen-year-olds in America had been diagnosed with ADHD at some point in their lives so far, representing a steady rise since the 1990s.[4] Over a third of foster children in the United States use a psychotropic medication, and over 40 percent of that group use three or more such medications at the same time.[5]

Advertising and marketing help keep the consumption of medication high and rising. Researchers exploring the effects of direct-to-consumer advertising on patient and physician behavior found that in 1995, 3 percent of physician office visits by youth aged fourteen to eighteen resulted in a prescription for a psychiatric drug; in 2001, 8 percent of office visits did. Their data points frame the year 1997, when direct-to-consumer advertising of prescription drugs was first allowed.[6]

While data reflecting population-level use of pharmaceuticals roll out slowly, the latest analyses suggest that SSRI use among children under eighteen underwent a modest decline, around 15 percent, in the few years after the FDA mandated that a black-box warning label about the risk of suicidal behaviors in children be placed on SSRIs' packaging in 2004. (There was a concomitant small rise in the number of children treated with talk therapy.)[7] It remains to be seen whether these changes last, and whether they are part of a larger move away from psychopharmaceutical use in children, or merely a sign that the medication frontier has moved elsewhere.

If sales figures are a guide, that frontier may now consist of a family of drugs called atypical antipsychotics, which became the top-selling drug class by revenue in the United States in 2009. (Though they are used by many fewer people than use SSRIs, they are much more expensive.)[8] Over half a million children and adolescents in the United States now take atypicals,[9] whose brand names include Abilify, Zyprexa, Risperdal, and Seroquel. In children with severe behavioral problems, atypicals—which are also known as "major tranquilizers"—are often prescribed to augment the stimulants used to treat ADHD.[10] The use of atypicals in children and teens is controversial because the drugs cause pronounced weight gain, increase the risk of diabetes, and can cause muscle spasms, twitches, and tics that may or may not go away even after the patient stops the drugs.[11] In spite of these dangers, antipsychotic medications have found a use in children because the drugs "can settle almost any extreme behavior, often in minutes, and doctors have few other answers for desperate families."[12]

The companies that make atypical antipsychotics have promoted their use in young patients. A *New York Times* investigation into public records in Minnesota found that over a third of the state's psychiatrists accepted payments from drug makers, that an increase in payments over recent years was associated with a ninefold increase in atypical antipsychotic prescriptions for children on the state's Medicare rolls, and that the doctors who accepted the most money from the manufacturers of atypicals appeared to prescribe those drugs most often.[13]

Consumers in the United States use far more psychiatric medication than people in many other countries. Rates of antidepressant use by youth in the United States are between three and fifteen times higher than in continental Europe,[14] and the

United Kingdom has been slower to embrace antidepressants for young people as well.[15] Antidepressant use by youth less than doubled through the 1990s in some places in Europe, while in the United States it increased sixfold from the late 1980s to the mid-1990s, then doubled again, and again.[16] Polypharmacy, the practice of prescribing a second or third psychotropic medication to augment the benefits or combat the side effects of a first, is rare outside of the United States, but it is prevalent and rising in popularity here.[17] The reasons for these discrepancies are not definitively understood, but they likely include variation in cultural beliefs about the point at which a behavior becomes a pathology, and also the influence of direct-to-consumer pharmaceutical advertising, which is not currently permitted in any European country.

Whatever the total constellation of reasons, psychiatric medications have become a part of us: so much so that scientists collecting samples downstream from a wastewater treatment plant in North Texas in 2003 discovered metabolites of Prozac and other antidepressants in every single fish they tested.[18]

In 2013, the American Psychiatric Association is expected to release the next edition of the diagnostic manual, DSM-5. In keeping with tradition, the book will have expanded to include new categories of disorders. For the first time, a number of diagnoses will include severity scales, making it possible to have certain disorders in mild, moderate, or severe degrees. While I appreciate the move away from the binary, the skeptic in me expects the possibility of having a "mild" case of something to result in further diagnostic-bracket creep, more diagnoses, more prescriptions, and ever-greater shrinkage of that beleaguered old category of normal.

People who defend the biomedical turn in psychiatry often claim that this move has been vital in reducing the stigma that's associated with mental illness. In the past, the story goes, people with depression and other serious mental disorders were viewed not as ill but as weak of character and were shamed or told unhelpfully to "snap out of it." Today, thanks to the push to see mental illnesses as legitimate, physical diseases, those who suffer are accorded the respect and care that is due them as people with a true affliction. There is much that is valid in this account. Mental health awareness has risen in recent decades. Several of the people I interviewed felt that they'd benefited personally by the chance to think of their problems as a kind of disease, reducing the attached stigma. The popularization of the idea that depression is an organic disorder may have given many people, for the first time, a way to talk about mental and emotional problems at all.

Yet the stigma question isn't as simple as it's often made out to be. What's been happening over the last few decades is more than just a removal of stigma from cases of mental illness that were once stigmatized, an unshaming of the previously shamed. By now, a troop of social scientists, journalists, and other observers have documented the ways that pharmaceutical companies actively "market" diseases, to doctors and the public alike (a feat they achieve by such means as funding public awareness campaigns and screening days, bankrolling patient-advocacy groups, and running educational retreats for doctors), and then tout their products as the means to treat these newly publicized ailments.[19] Drug companies that encourage us to perceive ever wider swaths of experience as mental illnesses aren't white knights waging a noble war to remove stigma from horribly stigmatized diseases.

Instead these companies are creating stigma* with one hand before they profitably remove it with the other. In carving out new territory for illness, they are stigmatizing what hadn't been before, and then—voilà!—declaring that the illnesses they've defined are real and, therefore, should not be stigmatized. With one gesture, they sicken us; with another, they turn around and remind us magnanimously that it isn't our fault that we are all so mentally ill—and ask us, by the way, whether we'd like to buy some medicine.

IN MY INTRODUCTION I wrote that one of the stranger things about growing up is attaining an age where you can look back and actually perceive historical change as having happened during your lifetime. When I read, when I talk to my parents about their experiences and reflect on my peers' and mine, when I try to think about what's been different for us, I start to see my generation as one that is defined by mobility and choice. We were raised in an era of unprecedented consumer abundance: brought up to count on disposability, endless customization, and a hundred varieties of any item we might desire. We have also lived through a marked breakdown of social expectations, particularly the expectation of continuity. The patterns that structure behavior and define our life plans are fading, the benchmarks that once defined success becoming less relevant and less dependable. Consider these oft-repeated facts: thirty years ago, a man might expect to work for the same company for all his life, but many young millennials expect to change jobs, and even fields, every

* At root, the word *stigma* means a sign or a mark; Erving Goffman, the sociologist who popularized its use, used it to mean the taking on or imposition of an identity that marks its bearer as abnormal.

year or two. The average age of marriage is rising. The women of my generation were raised by their second-wave feminist mothers to believe that we can (and should) do it all—pursue careers, have families, take time for ourselves—but with little hard guidance about how it's supposed to be possible to fit it all in. Relationships come with fewer expectations: that they'll last, or of what is meant by "relationship" at all, and sex more often takes place outside of them. Our lives feel unscripted; we are re-writing the roles from scratch. The erosion of expectations is freeing, but it can also generate a kind of panic, as it does for the high-achieving students Joseph Davis described, whose inability to conceive of definite goals for their ambition leads to a dizzying and constant feeling that they haven't achieved *enough*. We are moving and experimenting more, accumulating less. There's nothing holding us down.

There's nothing holding us down.

I remember reading, when I was thirteen or so, a lifestyle article in the newspaper about how people in their twenties were living together in shared rental houses. The article described this phenomenon as if it were new and fascinating, which is funny to me now, but what made it memorable then were the descriptions of the house and the lives of the people inside it. Rambling hallways, communal meals, good music on the stereo, funky jobs, interesting conversation late into the night—the piece painted a vivid picture of young adulthood as a promised land of easy community and bohemian good times, and I read it with a mounting sense of impatience for the day I'd be old enough to join the fun.

Do I need to tell you that it wasn't always like that? The period after college, in particular, was a hard time for me, as it is for many. Aware of our advantages, my friends and I were surprised to find ourselves feeling so lost. The world seemed sharp-elbowed and mysterious, and real community was hard to locate. Sometimes I wonder whether one thing antidepressants have done in my time is to help underwrite this unprecedented historical invention, *one's twenties*, a long period of time in which we're permitted to explore, to not be settled down, to wander among the social and economic and physical landscapes of our country, trying to find a place for ourselves. This wandering is a privilege and often fun, but it is also difficult. Maybe it would not be so psychologically taxing if it were better defined, if its meaning were somewhere, in some way, clearly laid out for us. But it is not. We must each decide or work out what it means for ourselves; we must draw our own maps. It's hard to travel without a map, to wander. My sense is that some of us are better equipped, by constitution, for this wandering than others. Perhaps antidepressants are in part a technology that helps to make it supportable for the rest. Maybe they are capitalism's answer for some of the things that capitalism doesn't supply well: warmth, connection, and a diffuse sense—in a world of limitless possibility and little in the way of tradition—of rightness.

There's at least some evidence that I'm not inventing this sense that life has grown more unstable in recent years. Not long ago I was arrested by an American Psychological Association press release headline that screamed, "Average Child Today Is as Anxious as Average Child Mental Patient in the 1950s." The studies it referenced found that American children and college students alike display significantly more trait anxiety today than they did sixty years ago. The change correlates highly with a significant nationwide dip in the level of social embeddedness (as measured by factors like the prevalence of divorce, the percentage of people living alone, and how much individuals report trusting others), and a rise in the level of perceived overall threat (including factors like crime, and the fears of environmental degradation and nuclear war) over the last sixty years. "Societies with low levels of social integration produce adults prone to anxiety," the researcher wrote in her conclusion, noting that anxiety is a factor that predisposes people to depression. "Until people feel both safe and connected to others," she observed, "anxiety is likely to remain high."[20]

If our aggregate bad feelings really are in part the product of social disconnection, it is ironic that the remedy we've embraced is itself a disconnected one. Depression can be thought of as a crisis in one's ability to feel close and connected to others. But as medication becomes the standard of treatment for emotional disorders, human contact becomes less and less a part of the cure. As society grows less embedded, mental health care becomes less embedded too; in this generation, for the first time, the professionals in our society who are assigned to handle human emotional pain are often assigned to handle the emotional pain of 1,400 humans at once. And it's not just doctors that patients are disconnected from. As a cure, there's something a little pyrrhic about antidepressants; in order to obtain the relief that they offer, you have to consent to the premise that your pain is irrational. In both senses, antidepressants underscore the feeling of aloneness that they are supposed to mitigate.

It is easy to take a pill. It's forbiddingly difficult to remake society in a healthier image. It is also easy to take the flashy argument that mental illness consists of nothing more than being "sane in an insane world" too far. Mental illness is real, and medication benefits millions of people. If one thing emerged from the conversations I had for this book, it's a conviction that people who are treating an emotional problem do best when the treatment they use is the one they desire and believe will work. It is a powerful thing to talk to someone who uses a medication that they know helps them. If antidepressants impacted my generation by teaching us that we have some recourse to feeling fruitless misery, then they have done us a real and lasting benefit. But it is important for us to hold onto an awareness that there's more that goes into how we feel than the configuration of chemicals in our own brains. There is value in pushing back against the message—because it's so well-capitalized and comes out so loud—that suffering and sadness are always signs of disorder, or that there is nothing to be said for understanding them in any other way.

In themselves, antidepressants are a neutral technology. But as products that are sold to us, they arrive along with stories about how we ought to feel, and why we feel the way we do. It is in pharmaceutical companies' best interest that we feel confused about what is normal, and that we err on the side of assuming that any given problem could be a sign of a mental disorder. We need to remain aware of what these stories are, and continue to ask whether they are true and whether they serve our own best interests too. A simplified version of the biomedical model of mental illness can hurt us when it is carried too far into the way we think about life. The messages that come with medication become damaging when they begin to collapse the distinction between living free of mental illness, and living meaningfully or well—replacing a bigger conversation about our goals and values as individuals and as a society with a circumscribed one that revolves around illness and its saleable treatments, rather than the conditions for health. When the choice of whether or not to medicate fills parents with guilt no matter what they select; when our preoccupation with psychopathology makes negative emotional states more distressing because we fear excessively that they may be signs of a serious problem; when we accept the chemical-imbalance story as an invitation not to think critically about how the environments we live in and the choices we make also contribute to how we feel, the prevalence of medication has begun to create background noise, a cacophony of worry and mystified expectations that distracts us from the real tasks of living, and actually makes it harder to grow up.

While some of us will need medication, or want it, we all need things that medication can't provide—things we shouldn't overlook in our enthusiasm for easily classified problems and quick, high-tech solutions. We need things that can't be commodified or manufactured, that can't be rendered more efficient, and that will never make any company rich. In our society, with its glistening surfaces, we all need reality checks. We need to talk to each other, as honestly as we can. We need help sorting out what's worthwhile from what isn't, what makes us feel good from what makes us feel bad. We need the comfort of feeling like we're not alone. We need meaningful work and real rest, or at least the hope of these. We need connection and love. And we need to learn, by trial and error, how to take care of ourselves.

Adults need to remember how much they can help, how much young people still need them. Once in a while, young people need an adult to notice when something is really wrong, to intervene and give a medical problem the dignity of a medical name. Without exception, they need grown-ups to pay attention, to listen and hear, and to set examples, not of TV-personality perfection, but of actual, struggling adulthood. They need someone who can walk the fine line between looking out for real trouble and speaking the age old, unmarketable words for which there is no substitute: *I know it hurts* and *Trust me, it's going to get better in time.*

NOW AND THEN, somebody asks me if I think I was *really depressed*, back in college. Of course I've asked myself the same thing. It is hard to know how to answer the question. It happened a long time ago now, and it's not easy to piece together the memory of an emotion after the fact. I think the only fair answer, though, is "yes." I was upset, to a degree so pronounced and different that it seemed to demand its own name. I don't know whether my upset was caused by biological factors or external ones, but the only plausible answer would seem to be a combined one: I was depressed because of a mysterious totality of forces, the contribution of my genes and neurons joining together with my life history, catalyzed by the things I was going through at the time.

Implicit in this question, "Were you really depressed?" is the question, "So, are you glad you took antidepressants?" That one is tougher to answer. Sometimes I catch myself wishing it had never happened. It's easy to fantasize about the ways my life could have been better without them: maybe I'd have stayed as serious about writing as I was in high school. Maybe if Zoloft hadn't killed my sex drive, things would have worked out differently with my college boyfriend, Jeff. Maybe, with all the time and energy I spent fretting about whether or not I was really myself on antidepressants, I'd have done something else, developed an interest that was more wholesome or outward-looking. On the other hand, I can't know whether things would have been worse. Maybe I'd have dropped out of school. Maybe I would have muddled through but had less fun, achieved less, not distinguished myself as much. Maybe I would have taken fewer risks in my life after graduation; maybe I'd have clung more, and maybe that would have been bad for me.

"What if" is an impossible game to win. I can't change the past, and I am happy with where I've ended up. So I say that no, I'm not sorry I used antidepressants. I am sorry, though, about how patchily I was supervised, especially at the beginning. I am sorry that I received medication first and psychotherapy only a long time after. Most of all, I'm sorry for how thoroughly I absorbed the message that came along with antidepressants, the one about having a sick brain. Antidepressants had been prescribed to me, as I took it, because I was crazy, because I felt things that didn't make any sense. That suggestion sank in deeply and lasted a long time, hollowing me out underneath the layer of brightness and confidence that the medication imparted. It made me think less of myself, kept me from noticing all the sense I did make, and enforced a tendency to underestimate my own strengths and overestimate the strengths of others that had been part of the problem from the very beginning.

When I think back to that time, it seems to me that one thing I needed was a message almost completely different from the one that antidepressants delivered. Instead of being told that my feelings were meaningless mutations, I needed some help identifying what those feelings really were. I needed to be told that I wasn't the only person to have them. I needed to hear that I could be excited about college but still miss home, that I could miss home but not be a wimp. Just as the best thing to do when you're losing control of your car on an icy road is to make the counterintuitive move of steering into the skid, I needed someone to tell me that it was all right to be upset, that I could even steer into it a little bit—that it was likely I would feel better soon and that if I didn't, there were other things we could try.

SOMETIMES, IN MY imagination, I travel back to Sam's office. I play our first meeting over again, but I make it go differently. Our conversation starts out the same: she asks me what's wrong, and I cry, and tell her. But then, instead of reaching for her pad, she talks to me. She tells me that moving all the way across the country for school is hard. I listen to her, swabbing at my eyes, interested and slightly incredulous. She asks about my life and tells me that it's good that I've made friends, good that I seem to be doing well in classes. I choke out the story of Brendan, and she remarks that even if I can't see it, it seems to her likely that he has some problems of his own. She tells me that in her opinion, I'm making a pretty decent transition, and by the time she says it, my breath is flowing in and out of my chest more smoothly. She advises me to go away for a few days, to try to take it easy on myself. Spend time with friends, keep her number nearby, call her if I need to. I thank her, she opens the strange double door of her office, and I clatter down her stairs and tumble out into the brightness of the day.

This too is a fantasy. I can't know whether it would have made the difference, whether I would have revived in a couple of days and never gone back. Maybe I wouldn't have recovered, and we'd have started medication eventually anyway; or if not then and with Sam, it would have happened somewhere else. In either case, having such a conversation would have given me a different perspective on my problems from the one offered by drugs. It would have made those problems seem less strange and disturbing. And it might have planted much earlier a seed of the compassion for myself and the acceptance of vulnerability that ultimately made feeling bad so much easier to deal with, and that in the end it took me a long time to learn.

SEVERAL YEARS AGO, when I first started to get serious about writing this book, I was thinking intently about what it means to grow up. Over the course of a few months, I kept getting involved in the same conversation with different friends. We were all in our late twenties, and we remarked to one another that life felt different than it had just a few years before. We noticed it in ourselves and in each other too. People still went through rough times: they lost jobs and had breakups; some years and seasons were better than others. But we all agreed on one thing—no one seemed to be falling apart the way they had with regularity, in college and directly after.

Neuroscientists say that the brain keeps developing until we reach age twenty-five, that the circuits that produce fear and anxiety grow less excitable. Maybe that explains it: perhaps we'd finally myelinated our prefrontal cortices and were reaping the rewards. Or maybe we'd gotten used to the workings of the real world at last, and were gratefully watching our quarter-life crises fade into the rearview. I don't know what it was. All I knew was that I felt like I'd finally crawled up on dry land, and I was pleased and comforted that my friends seemed to be doing the same.

Looking back, I have no sophisticated explanation for the change. I think what happened was, quite simply, that we grew up.

I don't want to exaggerate the luxuries of this new place. Sometimes there are earthquakes. Sometimes the fog rolls in and stays for weeks. But it's fertile land, and arable too. It feels like a place where you can get some living done. While the storms aren't over, they do feel different now. And I'm confident in a way that I couldn't have imagined years ago of my ability to weather them.

Maybe you know this feeling, this place. Maybe you see it, up ahead, as a promise. I want to tell you that you'll get here too. Medication won't prevent you from making the trip, but it won't get you here on its own. You will get here by living, by engaging with the world, by loving and fighting and making mistakes, by picking yourself back up and trying again. You'll do it by taking support where you can—from medicine, from the people around you, from your interests and beliefs. If you are lucky, you'll find a guide who will help by listening to you and sharing the story of her own way across. The trip won't always be comfortable, but it will feel real, unique, and yours.

Maybe you are here already. If so, maybe you have experienced how, on a good day, the breezes change direction, and the feeling in the air shifts a little. The voices inside that once asked "Who am I?" quiet down, and into the silence a different, but related voice says softly, "Here you are. What will you do?"

ACKNOWLEDGMENTS

Many people helped in the making of this book. On the professional side, I'd like to thank my agent, Eva Talmadge; Allison Lorentzen; Suzanne Rindell; Emma Sweeney; Shelly Perron; and my editor, Michael Signorelli, who saw the project through with a winning blend of wisdom, clear-headedness, and good humor.

I am immensely grateful to everyone who took a chance on talking with me about their personal experiences, as well as to the psychiatrists, psychologists, and academics who shared their expert perspectives, both those whose words are captured in the book and those whose input provided valuable background—the latter group including Gabrielle Carlson, Joe Hewitt, Bradley Lewis, Sue Marcus, Benedetto Vitiello, and Julie Zito.

For answering questions, providing leads, and other acts of research largesse, I thank Andrew Boyd, Benjamin Cohen, Christina Dunbar-Hester, Andrew Lakoff, Jacks McNamara, Mark Olfson, Ken Paul Rosenthal, Lauren Russo, Nikhil Swaminathan, and Virginia Vitzthum; and at the U.S. CDC, Sheila Franco, Amy Bernstein, Richard Niska, and Jill Ashman. I also thank Rachel Prentice, whose course at Cornell first helped me discover my fascination with pharmaceutical advertising.

For places to work, I thank Jay Barksdale and the New York Public Library; Stephanie Harad and Anne Hinton; and the Sharpe and Towns families, which each put on a truly formidable DIY writer's retreat.

Close to home, I sing the praises of Jared Greenfield, Jessica Stults, and Alison Towns for their smart manuscript reading; Anna Bond, Stephanie H., and Meg McIntyre, my family of friends, for helping in ways concrete, ineffable, and every conceivable gradation in between; Sarah Jackson; Jesse Kraai; and with special honor, Susan Sharpe, whose encouragement, care, and incisive attention to the text were essential to the book, and its writer too. Thank you, thank you, thank you.

NOTES

INTRODUCTION

1. Olfson and Marcus, 848.
2. Ibid., 848.
3. National Center for Health Statistics. *Health, United States, 2010*, 19.
4. Gu et al., 5.
5. Ibid.
6. National Center for Health Statistics. *Health, United States, 2010*, 19.
7. Kirby.
8. Olfson and Marcus, 851.

2: A SHORT HISTORY OF MEDICATION

1. Laurence, 1.
2. Ibid.
3. World Health Organization, web.
4. Stewart et al.
5. Greenberg, 183.
6. Healy, *The Antidepressant Era*, 53.
7. Ibid., 47.
8. Ibid., 58.
9. Ibid., 47.
10. Ibid., 43.
11. Ibid., 46.
12. Ibid., 52.
13. Ibid., 54.
14. *New York Times*, April 7, 1957, "Science Notes: Mental Drug Shows Promise," 86.

15. Healy, *The Antidepressant Era*, 116.
16. Luhrmann, 236.
17. Healy, *The Antidepressant Era*, 61.
18. Ibid.
19. Ibid.
20. Ibid., 154.
21. Horwitz and Wakefield, 168–69.
22. Ibid.
23. "Professor Joseph Schildkraut." *Times* (London).
24. Luhrmann, 213.
25. Healy, *The Antidepressant Era*, 66.
26. Luhrmann.
27. Manners, 79.
28. Greenberg, 260.
29. Manners, 79.
30. Luhrmann, 223.
31. Horwitz and Wakefield, 85.
32. American Psychiatric Association. *Diagnostic and Statistical Manual of Mental Disorders, Second Edition*, 40.
33. Healy, *The Antidepressant Era*, 38.
34. American Psychiatric Association. *Diagnostic and Statistical Manual of Mental Disorders, Third Edition*, 1.
35. Healy, *The Antidepressant Era*, 167.
36. Manners, 80.
37. Healy, *The Antidepressant Era*, 168.
38. Pfizer, Inc.
39. Carlat, 40–43.
40. Kirsch.
41. Horwitz and Wakefield, 169.
42. Kirsch, 96–97.
43. Horwitz and Wakefield, 188.
44. Luhrmann, 228.
45. Curtis, "The Lonely Robot."
46. Kirn.

3: STARTING OUT

1. Karp, 57.
2. Stutz.

4: DECADE OF THE BRAIN

1. Paxil commercial.
2. Bush, George H. W.

3. Chocano.
4. Elson and Horowitz.
5. Elmer-DeWitt et al.
6. Ibid.
7. "Rasagiline," MedlinePlus.
8. Critser, 6.
9. Kaiser Family Foundation. "Impact of Direct-to-Consumer Advertising on Prescription Drug Spending," 4.
10. Kaiser Family Foundation. "Public and Physician Views of Direct-to-Consumer Prescription Drug Advertising."
11. Ibid.
12. Goetzl.
13. Coupland, 27.
14. "Homer Badman." *The Simpsons.*
15. "The Sopranos." *The Sopranos.*
16. Dennis.
17. Albarn.
18. Jagger and Richards.
19. *Garden State.*
20. Kramer, 18.
21. Ibid., 10, 19.
22. Ibid., 15.
23. Ibid.
24. Ibid., 14.
25. Martel.
26. "Depression Hurts." Commercial.
27. O'Neal and Biggs.
28. Elliott, xvi.
29. Ibid., 35.
30. "Barb's Golfing Again." Commercial.
31. "Sue's Playing with Her Kids Again." Commercial.
32. Cymbalta commercial.
33. Celexa (Citalopram). *Rxstories.com.*
34. Ibid.

5: I'VE NEVER BEEN TO ME

1. Friedman.
2. Koplewicz, Harold. Telephone interview, June 17, 2008.
3. Mayo Clinic.

6: TWO RED CHAIRS

1. Harris, "Study Finds Less Youth Antidepressant Use."
2. Zito, "Off-label psychopharmacologic prescribing."
3. Ibid.
4. Marcus, interview.
5. Horney, 359.

7: FLIGHT OF THE DODO BIRD: EVALUATING THERAPY

1. Luhrmann, 204–5.
2. Greenberg, 300.
3. Luhrmann, 204.
4. Ibid., 206.
5. Greenberg, 300.
6. Ibid.
7. Ibid.
8. Luhrmann, 205.
9. Ibid., 206.
10. Quoted in Greenberg, 300.
11. Luhrmann, 207.
12. Ibid., 57.
13. Ibid.
14. Ibid., 75–76.
15. Freud and Jung, 10.
16. Luhrmann, 60.
17. Greenberg, 288.
18. Marcus, Sue. Personal interview, November 2, 2010.
19. Greenberg, 302.
20. Ibid.
21. Burns, 42.
22. Freud and Jung, 10.
23. The TADS Team.
24. Solomon, 103.
25. Olfson, "National patterns in antidepressant medication treatment," 848.
26. Horwitz and Wakefield, 185.
27. Ibid., 184.
28. Olfson, 854.
29. Harris, "Talk Doesn't Pay."
30. Whitaker, National Institute of Mental Health.

8: QUITTING

1. Cotman et al., 465–66.
2. Freeman.

3. Furihata et al.
4. Akbaraly et al., 411.
5. Galambos and Krahn, 21.
6. Ibid., 15.

10: THE NEXT GENERATION

1. Lewin.
2. American College Health Association, 31–32.
3. Barr et al., 24.
4. Gabriel.
5. University of California Office of the President, 3.
6. *Newsweek*, "Getting in Gets Harder."
7. Rimer.
8. Brooks, David, "The Organization Kid."
9. Schleider and Wong.
10. Lurie.
11. Davis, 38.
12. Davis, 45.
13. Davis, 48.
14. Ibid.
15. Glader.
16. Crawford.
17. Nolen-Hoeksema and Hilt.
18. Hilt and Nolen-Hoeksema.
19. Gilligan and Mikel Brown.
20. Mintz and Betz.
21. Lewin.
22. Sax.
23. For a fascinating, book-length account of the persistence of psychoanalytic thinking about women in the age of SSRIs, see Jonathan Metzl's *Prozac on the Couch*.

11: COMING OF AGE

1. Schwartz
2. Parens and Johnston, "Troubled Children."
3. NCHS Data Brief no. 42 (September 2010).
4. NCHS Data Brief no. 70 (August 2011).
5. Zito et al., "Psychotropic medication."
6. Thomas et al., 63.
7. Valluri et al., in *Medical Care*, 2010.
8. Wilson, "Child's Ordeal Shows Risk."
9. Ibid.

10. Zito, Julie. Telephone interview, April 8, 2011.
11. Zito, et al. "Off-label psychopharmacologic."
12. Harris, Carey, and Roberts.
13. Ibid.
14. Zito et al., "Antidepressant prevalence."
15. Healy, David. Telephone interview, October 25, 2010.
16. Zito, "Antidepressant prevalence."
17. Comer et al.
18. Walton, "Frogs, fish and pharmaceuticals."
19. On "marketing" diseases, see Greenberg's *Manufacturing Depression* and articles by Brendan Koerner and Paula Gardner.
20. Twenge, 1018.

BIBLIOGRAPHY

Akbaraly, Tasnime, et al. "Dietary pattern and depressive symptoms in middle age." *The British Journal of Psychiatry*. 195 (2009): 408–13.

Akinbami L. J., X Liu, P. N. Pastor, C. A. Reuben. "Attention deficit hyperactivity disorder among children aged 5–17 years in the United States, 1998–2009." NCHS Data Brief, No. 70. Hyattsville, MD: National Center for Health Statistics. 2011.

Albarn, Damon. "Country House." *The Great Escape*. Flood/Virgin Records, 1995.

Alonso, Silvia, et al. "Pollution by psychoactive pharmaceuticals in the rivers of Madrid metropolitan area (Spain)." *Environment International* 36 (2010): 195–201.

American College Health Association. "American College Health Association–National College Health Assessment (ACHA-NCHA II) Reference Group Data Report, Fall 2009." Baltimore: American College Health Association, 2010.

American Psychiatric Association. *Diagnostic and Statistical Manual of Mental Disorders (Second Edition)*. Washington, D.C.: 1968.

———. *Diagnostic and Statistical Manual of Mental Disorders (Third Edition)*. Washington, D.C.: 1980.

———. *Diagnostic and Statistical Manual of Mental Disorders (Fourth Edition): DSM-IV—4th ed., text revision. (Second Edition)*. Washington, D.C.: 2000.

"Barb's Golfing Again." Commercial. *American Journal of Psychiatry*. March 2000.

Barr, Victor, et al. "The Association for University and College Counseling Center Directors Annual Survey; Reporting Period: September 1, 2008, through August 31, 2009." Association for University and College Counseling Center Directors, 2010. (Accessed online as PDF.)

Brooks, David. "The Organization Kid." *The Atlantic*. April, 2001. Web. Accessed March 10, 2011.

Burns, David D. *Feeling Good: The New Mood Therapy*. Revised and Updated. (1980.) New York: Avon Books, 1999.

Bush, George H. W. Proclamation. "Decade of the Brain, 1990–1999, Proclamation 6158." Project on the Decade of the Brain. Library of Congress, n.d. Web. Accessed January 20, 2011.

Carlat, Daniel. "Mind over Meds: How I Decided My Psychiatry Patients Needed More from Me Than Prescriptions." *New York Times Magazine*, April 25, 2010: 40–43.

Carter, Gertrude, and Jeffrey Winseman. "A Prescription for Healing the Whole Student." *The Chronicle of Higher Education*. August 3, 2001. Web. Accessed March 5, 2011.

"Celexa (citalopram): Stories, Experiences, and Advice." *Rxstories.com*. Web. Accessed October 10, 2011.

Chaucer, Geoffrey. *Chaucer's Canterbury Tales, Volume 2*. Ed. Alfred W. Pollard. New York: Macmillan and Co., 1907.

Chocano, Carina. "We Think, Therefore We Diagnose." *Salon.com*. May 30, 2001. Web. Accessed January 3, 2011.

Comer, Jonathan, et al. "National Trends in Child and Adolescent Psychotropic Polypharmacy in Office-Based Practice, 1996–2007." *Journal of the American Academy of Child and Adolescent Psychiatry* 49:10 (October 2010): 1001–1010.

Cotman, Carl, et al. "Exercise builds brain health: key roles of growth factor cascades and inflammation." *TRENDS in Neurosciences* 30:9 (Sept 2007): 464–472.

Coupland, Douglas. *Generation X: Tales for an Accelerated Culture*. St. Martin's Griffin, 1991.

Crawford, Matthew. "Medicate U." *The American Interest Magazine*. September/October 2008. Web. Accessed February 16, 2011.

Critser, Greg. *Generation Rx: How Prescription Drugs Are Altering American Lives, Minds, and Bodies*. New York: Houghton Mifflin Harcourt, 2005.

Crystal, Stephen, et al. "Broadened Use of Atypical Antipsychotics: Safety, Effectiveness, and Policy Changes." *Health Affairs* 2009; 28(5): w770–w781.

Curtis, Adam. "The Lonely Robot." *The Trap: What Happened to Our Dream of Freedom*. BBC Two. March 18, 2007.

Cymbalta. Commercial. *YouTube.com*. Accessed May 14, 2011.

Davis, Joseph. "Adolescents and the Pathologies of the Achieving Self." *The Hedgehog Review*. Spring 2009: 37–49.

Dennis, Wendy. "Why Psychoanalysis Matters." *The Walrus*. September 2005. Web. Accessed December 28, 2010.

"Depression Hurts." Commercial. *Time*. July 21, 1997.

Dobbs, David. "The Science of Success." *The Atlantic*. December 2009. Web. Accessed November 6, 2010.

Donn, Jeff, et al. "Pharmawater II: Fish, wildlife affected by drug contamination in water." The Associated Press. N.D. Web. Accessed May 30, 2011.

Elliott, Carl. *Better Than Well: American Medicine Meets the American Dream*. New York: W. W. Norton, 2003.

Elmer-DeWitt, Philip, et al. "Depression: The Growing Role of Drug Therapies." *Time*, Monday, July 6, 1992. Web. Accessed January 8, 2011.

Elson, John, and Janice M. Horowitz. "Is Freud Finished?" *Time*. Monday, July 6, 1992. Web. Accessed January 8, 2011.

Emslie, Graham, et al. "Treatment for Adolescents with Depression Study (TADS): safety results." *Journal of the American Academy of Child and Adolescent Psychiatry*. December 2006, 45(12): 1440–55.

Finger, Stanley. *Minds Behind the Brain: A History of the Pioneers and Their Discoveries*. New York: Oxford University Press, 2004.

Foucault, Michel. *Technologies of the Self: A Seminar with Michel Foucault*. Ed. Luther H. Martin, et al. Amherst: University of Massachusetts Press, 1988.

Franklin, Deborah. "A Push for Colleges to Prioritize Mental Health." NPR.org. October 26, 2009. Accessed October 19, 2010.

Freud, Sigmund, and Carl Jung. *The Freud/Jung Letters*. Ed. William McGuire. Abridged ed. Princeton University Press, 1994.

Friedman, Richard. "Who Are We? Coming of Age on Antidepressants." *New York Times*. April 15, 2008. F5.

Furihata, Ryuji, et al. "Self-help behaviors for sleep and depression: A Japanese nationwide general population survey." *Journal of Affective Disorders* 130:1–2 (April 2011): 75–82.

Gabriel, Trip. "Mental Health Needs Seen Growing at Colleges." *New York Times*. December 19, 2010. Web. Accessed Feb. 16, 2011.

Galambos, Nancy, and Harvey Krahn. "Depression and anger trajectories during the transition to adulthood." *Journal of Marriage and Family* 70 (February 2008): 15–28.

Garden State. Dir. Zach Braff. Fox Searchlight, 2004.

Gardner, Paula. "Distorted packaging: marketing depression as illness, drugs as cure." *Journal of Medical Humanities* 24:1–2 (Summer 2003): 35–47.

"Getting in Gets Harder." *Newsweek*. January 3, 2008. Web. Accessed April 22, 2011.

Gilligan, Carol, and Lyn Mikel Brown. *Meeting at the Crossroads: Women's Psychology and Girls' Development*. Cambridge: Harvard University Press, 1992.

Glader, Paul. "From the Maker of Effexor: Campus Talks on Depression." *Wall Street Journal*. October 10, 2002.

Greenberg, Gary. *Manufacturing Depression: The Secret History of a Modern Disease*. New York: Simon & Schuster, 2010.

Goetzl, David. "Paxil." *Advertising Age*. June 26, 2000. Web. Accessed January 20, 2011.

Goode, Erica. "Study Finds More Children Taking Psychiatric Drugs." *New York Times*. January 14, 2003. Web. Accessed May 30, 2011.

Gu, Qiuping, et al. "Prescription drug use continues to increase: U.S. prescription drug data for 2007–08." NCHS data brief, No. 42. Hyattsville, MD: National Center for Health Statistics, 2010.

Harris, Gardiner. "Antidepressants Seen as Effective for Adolescents." *New York Times*. January 2, 2004. Web. Accessed Feb 21, 2011.

———. "Talk Doesn't Pay, So Psychiatry Turns Instead to Drug Therapy." *New York Times*. March 5, 2011. Web. Accessed March 12, 2011.

———. "Study Finds Less Youth Antidepressant Use." *New York Times*. September 21, 2004. Web. Accessed Feb. 21, 2011.

Harris, Gardiner, Benedict Carey, and Janet Roberts. "Psychiatrists, Children and Drug Industry's Role." *New York Times*, May 10, 2007. Web. Accessed February 21, 2011.

Healy, David. "Shaping the intimate: influences on the experience of everyday nerves." *Social Studies of Science* 34:2 (April 2004): 219–45.

———. *The Antidepressant Era*. Cambridge: Harvard University Press, 1999.

Hilt, Lori, and Susan Nolen-Hoeksema. "The emergence of gender differences in depression in adolescence." In Susan Nolen-Hoeksema and Lori Hilt, eds., *Handbook of Depression in Adolescents*. New York: Routledge, 2008.

Hippocrates, Jones, and Withington. *Hippocrates*. Volume 4. Cambridge: Harvard University Press, reprinted 1959.

"Homer Badman." *The Simpsons*. Greg Daniels and Jeffrey Lynch. November 27, 1994. Television.

Horney, Karen. *Neurosis and Human Growth: The Struggle Toward Self-Realization*. New York: W. W. Norton, 1950. Reissued 1991.

Horwitz, Allan, and Jerome Wakefield. *The Loss of Sadness: How Psychiatry Transformed Normal Sorrow into Depressive Disorder*. New York: Oxford University Press, 2007.

Hsia, Yingfen, and Kathryn Maclennan. "Rise in psychotropic drug prescribing in children and adolescents during 1992–2001: a population-based study in the UK." *European Journal of Epidemiology* 24 (2009): 211–16.

Jagger, Mick, and Keith Richards. "Mother's Little Helper." *Aftermath*. Decca Records, 1966.

Kaiser Family Foundation. "Impact of Direct-to-Consumer Advertising on Prescription Drug Spending." Menlo Park, CA: 2003.

———. "Public and Physician Views of Direct-to-Consumer Prescription

Drug Advertising." KFF.org. May 6, 2008. Web. Accessed January 20, 2011.

Karp, David. *Speaking of Sadness: Depression, Disconnection, and the Meanings of Illness*. New York: Oxford University Press, 1997.

Kirby, James. "Explaining racial and ethnic differences in antidepressant use among adolescents." *Medical Care Research and Review* 67:3 (June 2010): 342–63.

Kirn, Walter. "Living the Pharmaceutical Life." *Time*. September 29, 1997. Web. Accessed May 13, 2011.

Kirsch, Irving. *The Emperor's New Drugs: Exploding the Antidepressant Myth*. New York: Basic Books, 2010.

Koerner, Brad. "First, You Market the Disease . . . Then You Push the Pills to Treat It." *The Guardian* (UK). Tuesday, July 30, 2002.

Koplewicz, Harold. *More Than Moody: Recognizing and Treating Adolescent Depression*. New York: Perigee, 2002.

Kramer, Peter. *Listening to Prozac*. Revised Edition. New York: Penguin, 1997.

Laurence, William L. "Wide New Fields Seen for TB Drug, Including Aid to Narcotics Addicts." *New York Times*. July 5, 1952.

Lewin, Tamar. "Record Level of Stress Found in College Freshmen." *New York Times*. January 26, 2011. Web. Accessed March 5, 2011.

Luhrmann, T. M. *Of Two Minds: The Growing Disorder in American Psychiatry*. New York: Alfred A. Knopf, 2000.

Lurie, Julia. "Everyone's Battle: Confronting College Depression." *Huffington Post*. January 26, 2011. Web. Accessed February 22, 2011.

Manners, Steven. *Super Pills*. Vancouver: Raincoast Books, 2006.

Martel, Huguette. "If they had Prozac in the nineteenth century." Cartoon. *The New Yorker*, November 8, 1993: 92.

Mayo Clinic. "Depression (Major depression)." *Mayoclinic.com*. Web. Accessed October 10, 2011.

Mennigen, et al. "Waterborne fluoxetine disrupts the reproductive axis in sexually mature male goldfish, *Carassius auratus*." *Aquatic Toxicology* 100:4 (November 15, 2010): 354–64.

Metzl, Jonathan. *Prozac on the Couch: Prescribing Gender in the Era of Wonder Drugs*. Durham: Duke University Press, 2003.

Mills, Mike. *Does Your Soul Have a Cold?* Film, 2007.

Mintz, L. B., and N. E. Betz. Prevalence and correlates of eating disordered behaviors among undergraduate women. *Journal of Counseling Psychology* 35 (1998): 463–71.

Mojtabai, Ramin, and Mark Olfson. "National trends in psychotropic medication polypharmacy in office-based psychiatry." *Archives of General Psychiatry* 67:1 (2010): 26–36.

National Center for Health Statistics. *Health, United States, 2010: With Special Feature on Death and Dying.* Hyattsville, MD. 2011.

———. *Health, United States, 2007: With Chartbook on Trends in the Health of Americans.* Hyattsville, MD: 2007.

National Institute of Mental Health. "Odds of Beating Depression Diminish As Additional Treatment Strategies Are Needed." Press release. November 1, 2006. Web. Accessed October 10, 2011.

Nolen-Hoeksema, Susan, and Lori Hilt. "Gender Differences in Depression." *Handbook of Depression*, 2nd Ed. I. H. Gotlib and C. L. Hammen, eds. New York: Guilford Press, 2009.

Olfson, Mark. "Assessing the effects of the antidepressant black box warning on depression management." *Medical Care* 45:11 (November 2010): i–iii.

Olfson, Mark, and Steven C. Marcus. "National patterns in antidepressant medication treatment." *Archives of General Psychiatry* 66:8 (August 2009): 848–56.

Olfson, Mark, et al. "National trends in the use of psychotropic medications by children." *Journal of the American Academy of Child and Adolescent Psychiatry* 45:5 (May 2002): 514–21.

O'Neal, Brandi, and Melanie Biggs. "Sequenced Treatment Alternatives to Relieve Depression (STAR*D): Patient Education Manual." Web. Accessed on May 14, 2011.

Parens, Eric, and Josephine Johnston. "Understanding the agreements and controversies surrounding childhood psychopharmacology." *Child and Adolescent Psychiatry and Mental Health* 2:5 (2008). Web. Accessed January 21, 2011.

———. "Troubled Children: Diagnosing, Treating, and Attending to Context." Special Report, *Hastings Center Report* 41:2 (2011): S1–S32.

Paxil. Commercial. *YouTube.com.* Accessed December 29, 2010.

Pfizer, Inc. "Causes of Depression." Zoloft.com. Accessed March 18, 2010.

"Professor Joseph Schildkraut." *Times* (London). August 4, 2006. Web. Accessed November 15, 2010.

PBS Frontline, "The Medicated Child." January 8, 2008.

"Rasagiline." MedlinePlus. National Institutes of Health. N.D. Web. Accessed January 4, 2011.

Rimer, Sara. "Today's Lesson for College Students: Lighten Up." *New York Times.* April 6, 2004. Web. Accessed January 14, 2011.

Sax, Linda. "College Women Still Face Many Obstacles in Reaching Their Full Potential." *Chronicle of Higher Education* 54:5, September 28, 2007, B46–B47. Web. Accessed March 10, 2011.

Schleider, Jessica, and Madrianne Wong. "Swarthmore's Culture of Silence: Addressing Mental Health on Campus." *(Swarthmore) Daily Gazette.* February 18, 2011. Web.

Schwartz, Barry. *The Paradox of Choice: Why More Is Less*. New York: Harper Perennial, 2004.

"Science Notes: Mental Drug Shows Promise," *New York Times*, April 7, 1957: 86.

Shorter, Edward. *Before Prozac: The Troubled History of Mood Disorders in Psychiatry*, Oxford: Oxford University Press, 2008.

Simoni-Wastila, Linda. "Gender and Psychotropic Drug Use." *Medical Care* 31:1 (January 1998): 88–94.

Solomon, Andrew. *The Noonday Demon: An Atlas of Depression*. New York: Scribner, 2001.

Stewart, Walter F., et al. "Cost of lost productive work time among U.S. workers with depression." *JAMA* 289:23 (2003): 3135–3144.

Storr, Anthony. *Freud: A Very Short Introduction*. New York: Oxford University Press, 2001.

Stutz, Bruce. "Self-Nonmedication." *New York Times Magazine*. May 6, 2007. Web. Accessed March 10, 2010.

"Sue's Playing with Her Kids Again." Commercial. *American Journal of Psychiatry*. June 2000.

"The Sopranos." *The Sopranos*. David Chase. January 10, 1999. Television.

The TADS Team. "The Treatment for Adolescents with Depression Study (TADS): Long-Term Effectiveness and Safety Outcomes." *Archives of General Psychiatry* 64:10 (October 2007).

Thomas, Cindy Parks, et al. "Trends in the use of psychotropic medications among adolescents, 1994 to 2001." *Psychiatric Services* 57 (January 2006): 63–69.

Twenge, Jean. "The age of anxiety? Birth cohort change in anxiety and neuroticism, 1952–1993." *Journal of Personality and Social Psychology* 79:6 (2000): 1007–1021.

University of California Office of the President, "Student Mental Health Committee: Final Report."

Valluri, Satish, et al. "Impact of the 2004 Food and Drug Administration Pediatric Suicidality Warning on Antidepressant and Psychotherapy Treatment for New-Onset Depression." *Medical Care* 48:11 (November 2010): 947–54.

Vitiello, Benedetto, et al. "National estimates of antidepressant medication among U.S. children, 1997–2002." *Journal of the American Academy of Child and Adolescent Psychiatry* 45:3 (March 2006): 271–79.

Walton, Marsha. "Frogs, fish and Pharmaceuticals a Troubling Brew." CNN. CNN.com. November 14, 2003. Web. Accessed May 30, 2011.

Watters, Ethan. *Crazy Like Us: The Globalization of the American Psyche*. New York: Free Press, 2010.

Whitaker, Robert. "The STAR*D Scandal: A New Paper Sums It All Up." *Psychologytoday.com*. Web. Accessed August 26, 2011.

Wilson, Duff. "Child's Ordeal Shows Risk of Psychosis Drugs for Young." *New York Times*. September 1, 2010. Web. Accessed October 18, 2010.

———. "Side Effects May Include Lawsuits." *New York Times*. October 2, 2010. Web. Accessed June 10, 2011.

World Health Organization. "Mental Health: Depression." WHO.com, n.d. Web. January 20, 2011.

Zito, Julie M., et al. "Off-label psychopharmacologic prescribing for children: history supports close clinical monitoring." *Child and Adolescent Psychiatry and Mental Health* 2:24 (2008). Web.

———. "Antidepressant prevalence for youths: a multi-national comparison." *Pharmacoepidemiology and Drug Safety* 15 (2006): 793–98.

———. "Psychotropic medication patterns among youth in foster care." *Pediatrics* 121:1 (January 1, 2008): e157-e163.